PHYSICIAN ENTREPRENEURS: THE QUALITY PATIENT EXPERIENCE

IMPROVE OUTCOMES, BOOST QUALITY SCORES, AND INCREASE REVENUE

Wendy Leebov, EdD
Foreword by Jeffrey I. Lasker, MD

Physician Entrepreneurs: The Quality Patient Experience—Improve outcomes, boost quality scores, and increase revenue is published by HCPro, Inc.

ISBN 978-1-60146-278-7

HCPro, Inc., provides information resources for the healthcare industry.

HCPro, Inc., is not affiliated in any way with The Joint Commission, which owns the JCAHO and Joint Commission trademarks.

Wendy Lebov, EdD Author
Elyas Bakhtiari, Editor
Rick Johnson, Executive Editor
Matt Cann, Group Publisher
Doug Ponte, Cover Designer
Jackie Diehl Singer, Graphic Artist

Leah Tracosas, Copyeditor
Darren Kelly, Books Production Supervisor
Paul Singer, Layout Artist
Susan Darbyshire, Art Director
Jean St. Pierre, Director of Operations

Advice given is general. Readers should consult professional counsel for specific legal, ethical, or clinical questions.

Arrangements can be made for quantity discounts. For more information, contact:

HCPro, Inc.
P.O. Box 1168
Marblehead, MA 01945
Telephone: 800/650-6787 or 781/639-1872
Fax: 781/639-2982
E-mail: *customerservice@hcpro.com*

HCPro, Inc. is the parent company of HealthLeaders Media.
Visit HCPro at its World Wide Web sites:
www.hcpro.com and *www.hcmarketplace.com*

09/2008
21499

Contents

About the Author

A passionate advocate for creating healing environments for patients, families, and the entire healthcare team, **Wendy Leebov, EdD** has 20 years of experience helping healthcare and human resources teams to provide care and service with compassion. During 20 years of service with the Albert Einstein Healthcare Network in Philadelphia, Wendy was most recently vice president of human resources. She also founded the Einstein Consulting Group, nationally respected for helping more than 300 healthcare organizations achieve service excellence and leadership effectiveness. Wendy received her bachelor of arts in sociology/anthropology from Oberlin College as well as her master's in education and doctorate in human development from the Harvard Graduate School of Education.

Leebov has written more than 12 books for healthcare leaders, including *Indispensable Health Care Manager, Achieving Impressive Customer Service, Service Excellence: The Customer Relations Strategy for Health Care,* and *Healthcare Managers in Transition.* She has also created many online toolkits, leadership toolkits, manuals, and articles.

For more information, visit *www.wendyleebov.com.*

Foreword

I know Wendy's work well. When I was president of Affiliated Pediatric Practices, and on the Board of Trustees of Partners Community Healthcare, Inc., we engaged her to help us develop and implement a long-term strategy to create legendary patient experiences in our 17 primary care pediatric practices. This was by far one of our most successful improvement efforts. Wendy's work was invaluable to us. Also, in my current role as Chief Executive Officer and Chief Management Officer of New England Quality Care Alliance, the physician network for Tufts Medical Center, I brought Wendy in to present at our provider conference. Our folks want her back!

Her strategies work. They helped us involve our teams, move toward effective patient-centered care, and position doctors to perform well on patient satisfaction surveys.

Wendy's book provides the same focus and attention to detail that makes her so terrific in person. She built on her years of experience to make available to physicians useful tools and tactics we can use to make our practices more successful—all by making the patient experience an exceptional one. The book is organized around the sections of the Consumer Assessment of Healthcare Providers and Systems (CAHPS) survey so it's also easy to find tools and information that help with CAHPS performance.

Her substantive section on the physician-patient relationship is not only a good reminder, it goes beyond platitudes and to identifies very specifically the communication fine points that help us connect to patients in ways that earn their respect and also improve outcomes.

Her chapter on maintaining high levels of patient experience while using an electronic health record (EHR) will be a big help to our providers, since EHR implementation has moved high on our agenda. Our providers will have easy-to-follow techniques that will make it possible to implement the EHR without it getting in the way of their interactions with patients. Also, her ample experience with office staff and all members of our teams really shows when she describes how to involve everyone in making the patient experience great.

Finally, the CD-ROM toolkit is a real find. There are many tools ready to use and this will save us time. These tools show exactly what to do to achieve a patient-centered culture and involve all staff in the process. While the array of tools may at first seem overwhelming, Wendy explains how to draw on them to develop a long-term approach that is manageable in a variety of settings.

Wendy's book and the CD-ROM provide an invaluable guide to making the patient experience a quality one and reaping the benefits in patient adherence and loyalty.

Jeffrey I. Lasker, MD, is CEO and CMO of the New England Quality Care Alliance.

Introduction

The Benefits of the Quality Patient Experience

As margins shrink and costs outpace revenue for most physicians, enhancing the patient experience is pivotal to your medical practice's success and profitability. Patient satisfaction plays an increasingly important role in the quest for accountability in healthcare—accountability to payers, purchasers, accrediting agencies, and even consumers. Improving patient satisfaction can benefit your practice in a multitude of ways.

Patient retention, loyalty, and growth

By providing consistently satisfying patient experiences, you win patients' loyalty and become their provider of choice. Your patients spread the word about your practice, which brings you even more patients. As people in your community shop around for doctors, you attract new patients via positive word-of-mouth from your current patients.

In addition to bettering your reputation in your community, improving patient satisfaction can also help you fare better with provider scorecard initiatives, which are proliferating to assist purchasers in their buying decisions. Recently, 28 large U.S. employers have adopted the "care-focused purchasing" approach that takes into account not claims data but outcomes, patient satisfaction, and efficiency in an effort to help employers and employees make more informed healthcare choices. Providing a quality patient experience may be the most effective growth strategy and marketing tactic your practice can pursue.

Success with accreditation and regulatory agencies

Agencies that accredit health plans scrutinize patient satisfaction data during the accreditation process. Health plans annually measure patient satisfaction as an external review and accreditation requirement of the National Committee for Quality Assurance, which instituted a member satisfaction survey as part of its Healthcare Effectiveness Data and Information Set quality standards as well as the Agency for Healthcare Research and Quality's (AHRQ) Consumer Assessment of Healthcare Providers and Systems (CAHPS) survey that measures the experiences of patients with their physicians and medical groups. The CAHPS Clinicians and Groups Survey is intended to bring transparency and standardization to the medical community, with results available to consumers, competitors, and employers through the National CAHPS Benchmarking Database.

Favored relationships with health plans

To become the plan of choice for consumers, health plans want to show high CAHPS scores to prospective customers. They want to retain members in their plan but know they defect when they are dissatisfied, so most have instituted several incentives or sanctions—all designed to encourage practices to enhance the patient experience. Common approaches include:

- Using feedback to drive improvement. Some health plans, such as the Harvard Pilgrim Health Plan, send patient satisfaction and clinical performance data back to capitated physician practices, along with comparative data from the rest of their respective networks. The intention: to trigger self-improvement efforts among physicians.

- Recredentialing. Other plans, such as Highmark, restrict the recredentialing of physician practices because of low scores, usually resulting in a practice receiving only a one-year, rather than a three-year, contract renewal.

- Offering financial incentives. With primary care physicians, many plans are using patient satisfaction data as the basis for bonuses or other financial incentives for practices with capitated payment contracts. Independence Blue Cross counts member satisfaction as 50% of primary care physicians' practice quality assessment score, which is used to calculate bonus payments, while some California plans give it a weight of 100% based on the mindset that healthcare is a service business.

The more satisfied your patients are with your practice, the greater negotiating power you have with payers.

Lower costs of doing business

By providing the exceptional patient experience, you also reduce the costs of doing business: Patients who are more satisfied with their experience are also less likely to file malpractice lawsuits. Given the direct relationship between patient satisfaction and likelihood to sue, you avoid losing time and money to malpractice litigation. You also create a more satisfying work climate for your staff, which in turn lessens costly staff turnover.

Reputation, pride, and satisfaction

In an atmosphere of consumer savvy and scrutiny, providing great patient experiences wins you and your practice an admirable reputation that results in widespread respect for you in your community. You build relationships with your patients that last. They trust you and partner with you in their care. Because they are more satisfied, they complain less. And all of this translates into greater job satisfaction and even greater pride in your contribution to people's health status.

Profitability

By providing an exceptional patient experience, you win favor from consumers, purchasers, accrediting agencies, and health plans that affect your practice's financial health directly. As a result of all of the factors described earlier, this translates into greater profitability.

Two invaluable benefits

By enhancing the patient experience, you strengthen your practice's performance on all of the factors described in the previous section, all while enjoying two additional benefits undoubtedly of ultimate value to you: improved outcomes and greater job satisfaction.

Improved outcomes and healthier patients: While reaping the benefits of the great patient experience, your practice will also achieve optimal health outcomes with your patients. They will be less anxious during their visits and communications with you and your team, and you will have more success eliciting needed information from them and engaging them in decisions that affect their health. Because of greater trust, they will be more likely to take their medications as directed and follow through on their care plans. All of this adds up to healthier patients.

Greater job satisfaction: All of these benefits lead to fewer frustrations and complaints, less stress, more engagement with your patients, and more satisfying relationships with patients, families, and your staff. You'll have the added benefits of a financially healthy practice and less stress.

CAHPS and accountability

Sponsored by the AHRQ, the CAHPS Survey for Clinicians and Groups assesses patients' experiences with their physicians and makes the results, which compare providers, available to patients, employers, health plans, and other purchasers of physicians' services. The Clinicians and Groups Survey, developed with significant input from patients, providers, health plans, and purchaser communities, provides important information about what patients and purchasers want from physicians and medical practices.

This survey is comprised of three instruments:

1. Adult Primary Care Questionnaire
2. Adult Specialty Care Questionnaire
3. Child Primary Care Questionnaire

In all three versions, there is a core questionnaire that is the same. It addresses three domains:

1. Getting appointments and healthcare when needed
2. How well doctors communicate
3. Courteous and helpful office staff

Each version includes additional questions tailored to it.

To help your practice thrive in this environment of increasingly available comparative data and accountability, this book explores key factors in each of the three identified domains and presents information and practical tools that will help you enhance your patients' experience and improve patients' perceptions of your practice.

Clinician and Group Core Survey Questions

Getting appointments and healthcare when needed	
Q6	In the past 12 months, when you phoned this doctor's office to get an appointment for care you/[your child needed right away, how often did you get an appointment as soon as you thought you/[your child] needed it?
Q8	In the past 12 months, when you made an appointment for a check-up or routine care [for your child] with this doctor, how often did you get an appointment as soon as you/[your child] thought you needed it?
Q10	In the past 12 months, when you phoned this doctor's office during regular office hours, how often did you get an answer to your medical question that same day?
Q12	In the past 12 months, when you phoned this doctor's office after regular office hours, how often did you get an answer to your medical question as soon as you needed?
Q13	Wait time includes time spent in the waiting room and exam room. In the past 12 months, how often did you/[your child] see this doctor within 15 minutes of your/[his or her] appointment time?
How well doctors communicate	
Q14	In the past 12 months, how often did this doctor explain things [about your child's health] in a way that was easy to understand?
Q15	In the past 12 months, how often did this doctor listen carefully to you?
Q17	In the past 12 months, how often did this doctor give you easy-to-understand instructions about taking care of these health problems or concerns?
Q18	In the past 12 months, how often did this doctor seem to know the important information about your/[your child's] medical history?
Q19	In the past 12 months, how often did this doctor show respect for what you had to say?

Clinician and Group Core Survey Questions

Q20	In the past 12 months, how often did this doctor spend enough time with you/[your child]?
Courteous and helpful office staff	
Q24	In the past 12 months, how often were clerks and receptionists at this doctor's office as helpful as you thought they should be?
Q25	In the past 12 months, how often did clerks and receptionists at this doctor's office treat you with courtesy and respect?
Overall rating	
Q23	Using any number from 0 to 10, where 0 is the worst doctor possible and 10 is the best doctor possible, what number would you use to rate this doctor?

Source: Items in the Reporting Composites and Overall Ratings for the CAHPS® Clinician & Group Survey- Core Questionnaires. Agency for Healthcare Research and Quality, Rockville, MD. December 2006.

CD-ROM Toolkit Instructions

The CD-ROM Toolkit contains tools and templates that you can use to build or strengthen your practice's culture so that everyone on your team contributes to patient-centered care and service.

You'll find here a description of how to use this toolkit along with a rich collection of tools in each of the following sections:

I: Observation and Feedback Tools
  - How to Do a Walk-through of Your Practice
  - The Quick Report Card
  - Post-Visit Phone Interview
  - Staff Meeting to Identify Staff Perceptions of Service Quality
  - Environment Audit

II: Tools to Enhance the Patient Experience in Everyday Situations
  - Great Greetings
  - Great Handoffs
  - Great Goodbyes
  - Presence
  - Acknowledging Feelings
  - Expressing Caring Nonverbally
  - Explaining Positive Intent

- Offering the Blameless Apology
- Giving the Gift of Positive Regard
- Using the Caring Broken Record

III: Tools for Staff Performance Management

- Great Customer Service: Hiring Tools
- Accountability Tools
- Employee Recognition Tools
- Flyers/Posters that Raise Staff Awareness
- Tools for Handling Delays and Waiting
- Tools that Ease Strain Related to Insurance and Money
- A Huge Variety of Scripts for Difficult Situations

Access and Continuity of Care

Of the 21 Consumer Assessment of Healthcare Providers and Systems (CAHPS) survey items that ask patients to evaluate their physician's practice, five are related to access. Access is pivotally important to your practice's success and to patient evaluations of their experience with your practice.

Access questions from CAHPS

1. Patient got appointment for urgent care as soon as needed
2. Patient got appointment for nonurgent care as soon as needed
3. Patient got answer to medical question the same day he or she phoned doctor's office
4. Patient got answer to medical question as soon as he or she needed when phoned doctor's office after hours
5. Patient saw doctor within 15 minutes of appointment time

Access to your practice shapes the patient experience even before the patient connects with a provider. Patients describe an obstacle course of phone calls not returned, telephone tag, long waits for appointments, jumping through insurance company hoops for precerts and referrals, voicemail hell, and automated answering systems that lead to nowhere—all just to connect to the provider or service they need. Such obstacles add anxiety to the substantial anxiety many patients already feel when they need to see a doctor or access healthcare services.

It's no wonder that people are joining telemedicine and concierge-style practices in droves, all because they want easy access. Services such as Doctor On Call that provide 24-hour phone access to a doctor for an annual membership fee are always springing up. And services like Consult-A-Doctor promise employers that they will reduce healthcare costs by providing access to licensed physicians by telephone or secure e-mail, and indeed such services have replaced up to 66% of doctors' office visits for their members. Instead of seeing their primary care physician for purely informational concerns and basic care, patients can reach a doctor on-call 24/7.

How Accessible Is Your Practice? 20 Questions

Complete this access audit to assess patients' access to your practice.

Practice Access: 20 Questions

	Never	Rarely	Half the time	Often	Always
1. When patients call the office, they reach the information or person they need without getting lost in voicemail or being placed on what seems like endless hold.					
2. When patients leave a message requiring a callback, someone from the practice calls back in a timely fashion.					
3. The provider has a system for preventing telephone tag when the patient is trying to connect.					
4. The patient can easily make an appointment.					
5. Except for rare situations, patients can see their own doctor.					
6. The patient can get a same- or next-day appointment.					
7. Office hours are convenient for students, elderly people, employed people, and families.					
8. If you have automated phone triage, the caller has the option to reach a live person.					
9. The patient can find the practice location without frustration.					
10. There is accessible parking or valet parking.					
11. Signs tell the patient where to go.					
12. The office is easily accessible for people with crutches, a wheelchair, or a cane.					
13. The office environment, furniture, and equipment are accessible to people regardless of age, size, or disability.					
14. The patient can reach the practice via e-mail.					

15. If the patient can reach the practice by e-mail, someone responds within 24 hours.					
16. The practice has 24/7 coverage.					
17. The practice staff helps patients secure referrals or precert paperwork when their insurance company requires it.					
18. Patients understand how to reach a doctor in emergency and nonemergency situations.					
19. Doctors in this practice have admitting privileges in respected, convenient hospitals.					
20. Patients perceive easy access as a strength of this practice.					

The higher your score, the better access your patients have to your practice. Each item with a moderate or low score reflects an opportunity to enhance access. Read on for opportunities to enhance access, and thereby the patient experience.

On the accompanying CD-ROM you'll find a variety of tools related to the material in Section I, including:

- How to Do a Walk-through of Your Practice
- The Quick Report Card
- Post-Visit Phone Interview
- Staff Meeting to Identify Staff Perceptions of Service Quality

1

The Practice Environment

When patients come for a visit, the ambience in your office affects their mood, anxiety level, and comfort. The physical environment, furniture, and equipment also have implications for access or, more pointedly, accessibility.

By consciously accommodating the diverse needs of your patient population, your office location, space, signage, and overall user-friendliness can reflect well on you and your practice, making it more inviting to patients and more satisfying for the people who choose to be your customers.

The juggling act

Your office space needs to be flexible enough to accommodate changing technology and procedure options. From the patient's perspective, the best location is accessible, convenient, and close to related services. From your clinical and nonclinical staff members' perspectives, your space needs to foster efficiency while at the same time ensuring privacy, confidentiality, sanitation, security, and comfort. It's a juggling act to consider the many specifications that make your environment optimal for both patients and your staff.

To determine strengths and improvement opportunities related to your office environment, have your staff—or better yet, a few patients, as well—complete the audit in Figure 1.1 to determine strengths and improvement opportunities of your office environment. You'll find that some improvement options will cost you nothing, while others have a cost but might merit a place on your "to do" list the next time you decide to invest in office improvements.

FIGURE 1.1 Environment Audit

Question	Yes	No
1. Is the name of your building obvious and easy-to-read from several angles (e.g., the road, the parking lot, etc.)?		
2. Is the parking area clearly marked, nearby, and well lighted?		
3. Is it easy and safe for someone to drop off a patient?		
4. Are the drop-off area, the main entrance, and route to your office barrier-free?		
5. Are there taxis available nearby, or a method for calling taxis as needed?		
6. Once people enter your building, is the way to your office clearly indicated?		
7. Is your reception desk positioned so that your staff members can quickly see people when they enter?		
8. Are work surfaces and equipment unrelated to registration hidden from the view of people in your reception area?		
9. Do you have no-glare lighting and no-glare coverings on counters and surfaces?		
10. Does your reception area have shelves, hooks, or closets for the personal items of patients and their companions?		
11. Do you provide specially designed areas conducive to reading, child's play, and conversation?		
12. Do you have a play area with toys/materials that are durable, safe, and usable by more than one child at a time?		
13. Does the waiting area have windows to the outside and to the hallway?		
14. If you have a television in the waiting area, is it positioned so that not everyone has to watch and hear it?		
15. Are chairs arranged so that people can choose to sit alone or in comfortably close groups, as they wish?		

FIGURE 1.1 Environment Audit (cont.)

16. Are your chairs comfortable for children, obese people, tall people, pregnant women, older people, and weak people?		
17. Are your exam and treatment rooms decorated in a way that is comfortable, colorful, and noninstitutional?		
18. Is there a phone available for patients and family members?		
19. Do people find your waiting area comfortable during a long wait?		
20. Is your waiting area upbeat and bright?		
21. Are patient education materials easily accessible to people who are waiting?		
22. Are trash receptacles available in your waiting area?		
23. Are easy-to-read clocks in reception and exam rooms?		
24. Do furniture arrangements facilitate eye contact between people talking with one another without barriers?		
25. Do you have private offices, cubicles or partitions that provide privacy?		
26. Do rooms where people undress have doors the patient can lock or ways the patient can indicate that the room is occupied and that they do not want to be disturbed?		
27. Is there a convenient bathroom and drinking water for people in the waiting area, as well as for patients who are gowned?		
28. Do you have a place for people to put their clothes and personal items when they undress, such as hooks, hangers, shelves, and hampers?		
29. Are exam and treatment rooms soundproof enough that people can't hear what's happening from one room to another?		
30. Do you have an extra chair in exam rooms for a family member or companion?		

FIGURE 1.1 Environment Audit (cont.)

31. Do you have comfortable furniture for obese people, such as sturdy open-arm chairs and firm sofas?		
32. Do you have body scales with a capacity of 300-plus pounds?		
33. Do you have exam tables accessible to all—that is, wide tables with adjustable heights?		
34. Do you have gowns large enough that patients of any size can avoid a struggle to cover themselves?		
35. Do you have step stools with handlebars?		
36. Are your floors clear of throw rugs or uneven seams that cause people with less-than-perfect eyesight to trip?		
37. Are the signs leading to and within your offices in colors visible to color-blind people?		
38. Are the signs leading to and within your offices in neat, large bold print for easy reading?		
39. Do you have nonslip floors?		
40. Are walkways clear?		
41. Is free wireless Internet available to people who are waiting?		
42. Are areas visible to people in the reception area free of clutter?		
43. Do the office acoustics both contain the noise level and make it easy for hard-of-hearing people to distinguish sounds?		
44. Do the doors in your office stay open long enough for people to enter and exit easily before they close?		
45. Do all areas appear clean?		

Five overarching office needs

Meeting the following five patient needs is paramount to providing an environment conducive to patient comfort and satisfaction:

1. **Wayfinding:** Patients will be stressed when they have any sort of problem finding or making their way to your office. Maps, transportation options, convenient parking, and clear signs and graphics are all important considerations to remove impediments and improve access.

2. **Physical comfort:** Chairs, lighting, room arrangements, furniture design, assistive devices and railings, smells, colors, textures, and noise all influence the patients' comfort level.

3. **Privacy and personal territory:** People appreciate the ability to control the extent to which they interact with others. The optimal environment caters to people with different preferences.

4. **Noise:** In *The Devil's Dictionary*, Ambrose Bierce defines noise as "a stench in the ear." Bothersome noise can interfere with relaxation, leads to irritability and anxiety, and even increase people's perception of pain. People expect to have peace and quiet in the doctor's office.

5. **Sense of security:** People want to know they are protected against slips, slides, and falls, and they want to be confident that equipment will hold them.

With so many factors to keep in balance, it's important to use the patient's experience as your compass to guide you in making facility improvements. Think about what your patients will see, feel, hear, and smell as you move through your practice. What will their frustrations be in the environment, and even during their trip to your office? Tuning in to the patient perspective is key to manipulating your office environment to heighten patient satisfaction so that everything about your office says to the patient "we care about you."

2

Easing Wait Times

Technological advances have destroyed what small tolerance people ever had for waiting. E-mail, voicemail, fax, FedEx, Priority Mail, instant messaging, high-speed Internet, and the like have changed consumer expectations: We want everything, and we want it now.

Waiting for appointments, waiting to see the doctor, waiting for results, waiting for a callback, waiting for an answer—all kinds of waiting in a medical practice irritate patients and can stir resentment toward your practice team. And a patient's growing impatience makes achieving and sustaining satisfaction more difficult. As consumers become understandably and increasingly demanding, speed has become a powerful competitive factor in patient satisfaction.

Opening access

Patients hate waiting to get an appointment, and in many practices the wait for an appointment is, from their viewpoint, outlandish. In recent years many practices have successfully reduced patient frustration through "open-access" scheduling, which makes it possible for a medical practice to provide appointments immediately or on the same day.

Same-day, advanced access, and *open access* are three terms for the scheduling model based on offering same-day appointments to all patients who call. The results: No long waits or delays in care, no triage, no deflecting patients to another-day appointment or another provider, and no stress from dealing with upset patients. The model has been proven time and time again to allow for faster attention to people's health issues, increased efficiency, and dramatic improvements in the patient experience, as patients no longer endure frustration about waiting for an appointment.

In my experience with various practices, their transitions to open scheduling have produced impressive benefits, including:

- Greatly reduced wait time for routine appointments
- Improved patient satisfaction with the appointment times they were able to get
- Increased percentage of patients who matched with their own physician
- Increased visit volume as a result of fewer no-shows and better efficiency
- Providers able to reduce their office hours per week

Sound like a panacea? In a way, it is, but note that there is no easy recipe for converting to open-access scheduling. Practice leaders need to tailor this kind of system to their unique circumstances.

The key is to ground your plan in a set of tested principles:

1. Measure, analyze, and understand your supply and demand. These need to be balanced; you will not be able to sustain open-access scheduling if demand for appointments typically exceeds supply. If you accept more patients than you can handle in a timely fashion, you must turn down appointments, which plays havoc with the patient experience.

2. Develop a short-term strategy to reduce your backlog to zero so you can begin your new scheduling system on a predetermined date. There's no getting around the fact that you will have to work harder than usual in the short-run to make the transition to your new system on your conversion date. But of course, after that, both patients and physicians reap ongoing benefits.

3. Decrease the number of queues by shrinking the variety of appointment types and durations available. A single appointment length works best. It's easier for staff to manage, simpler for patients, and physicians find themselves getting into a rhythm that helps them stay on time. Also, staff who schedule appointments don't have to say no to patients who need a certain appointment type because the right-size slots are full. When longer appointments are critical, staff can combine two of the generic appointment slots.

4. Develop contingency plans for those occasions when you have more demand than expected or less capacity than anticipated.

5. Fine-tune the demand by matching patients to their own physician, maximizing what is accomplished in a single visit, and adjusting the interval between visit and return visits.

6. Allow some prescheduling of appointments for clinical follow-up. That way, you keep control of the follow-up appointment instead of risking that the patient will not follow through. You can also load these appointments into the lower-volume times of the day and week, so there will be less demand for such appointment times.

7. Address the bottlenecks and constraints that tie up physician time. For instance, shift as much work as possible from the physician to other members of the team.

8. Develop an education strategy for patients and staff. Clarify the approach, emphasizing its benefits for them. If some patients still insist (and few do) on prescheduling an appointment, honor the patient's preference, selecting time slots in the early morning or latter part of the week—whenever your volume tends to be lowest.

When you have open-access scheduling, you reduce the wait, which greatly enhances the patient's experience. Patient satisfaction improves. Your patients are more appreciative, cooperative, and loyal. Staffers experience less stress and fewer patient complaints. Costs of care are lower. Revenues are enhanced. And you optimize clinical outcomes by providing "just-in-time" care to patients in need.

The psychology of waiting

When people are waiting, they often experience a lot of stress. You can reduce this stress by remembering and attending to the following principles:

1. **Anxiety makes waiting seem longer.** We need to figure out words and ways to reduce anxiety. For example, say to patients:

- "If you need to use the restroom, don't hesitate. You won't lose your turn."
- "If you need to contact someone about how long you'll be, you're welcome to use this phone or your cell phone."
- "Would you like to read a magazine?"

2. **Waits of uncertain length are harder to tolerate.** Too often, staff members say nothing to patients about the upcoming wait because they are embarrassed or they don't know how to estimate the time. Nevertheless, practices must write scripts that staff can use to advise patients of their waiting time. For instance, "The doctor will be able to see you within 20 minutes," or, "It can take up to four hours before the doctor can see you because some procedures take unexpectedly long periods of time."

3. **Waiting feels longer when you don't know the reason for the wait.** People sit there and stew when staff members don't explain why patients are kept waiting. Make regular updates by staff a routine, not an afterthought. "Mrs. Jones, I realize you've been waiting for nearly two hours. I'm really sorry. I want to explain and give you an update. We've had ambulances bring in trauma victims through another entrance. These people need a lot of our staff's attention because they are in life-or-death situations. I'm sorry this has created a long wait for you. At this point, I'm estimating that it could be another 90 minutes."

4. **People are much less tolerant when their wait feels unfair.** Let patients know why they're waiting longer than others. For example: "Mr. Hardy, I want to explain why some people who arrived after you might be taken before you. People in this area are here for three different services. You will be taken when the team that provides the specific service you came for is ready. In the meantime, some other services might be ready for the people here for those services. So they are taken before you."

5. **The more valuable the service, the longer a person is willing to wait.** This is no excuse for being callous about keeping people waiting. Just because they lack alternative providers or want *this* doctor or *this* service doesn't make it acceptable to perpetuate long waits. Fix the flow to reduce the delays out of respect for the patients, even if the delays aren't causing you to lose business.

6. **Preprocess waits feel much longer than in-process waits.** It's important to get the care process moving, even if there will be delays along the way. Many emergency departments do bedside registration, have staging areas, or have triage nurses initiate tests immediately so that the person can be in process right away, even though there might then be long delays. In outpatient areas, people have an easier time waiting in the exam room than they do in the reception area because they feel that at least they are *in process*.

7. **Waiting alone feels longer than waiting in a group.** It helps the time pass if family and friends can keep a patient company during any delays. If you have a policy that prevents family and friends from joining patients in the exam room, reconsider it. Figure out a way to make it possible for other people to be with the patient.

8. **Time goes faster when you're occupied than when you're bored.** When people don't have anything to do, wait time feels longer. We need to use our considerable creativity and find ways to keep people occupied while they wait.

9. **If people believe that you feel bad about inconveniencing them, they will be less angry with you.** Help the individuals on your team learn to sincerely apologize to patients and families when we keep them waiting, no matter whose fault it is.

Plan of action

Patients and families perceive timeliness as an indicator of your respect for them. Because of its extreme importance to patients and families and to the level of wear-and-tear on your staff, it pays to explore and institute improvements in timeliness. Here's a five-point plan for increasing respect for your patients' time.

1. **Speed up the process.** Eliminate or reduce delays through process and technology improvements. Examples include implementing quality improvement processes, eliminating redundancies, limiting the number of people a patient interacts with during the course of his or her visit, reducing the distances patients must travel through your facility during their visit, and locating all supplies, equipment, and forms at the caregivers' fingertips. Eliminate obsolete steps: Hold a staff contest to find elements of a process that no longer serve a function. Acquire tools (e.g., computers and equipment) that work faster. Conduct flow analyses and staff up at the logjam points.

2. **Remove the term "waiting room" from all signs, literature, and patient–staff interactions.** If patients must wait, provide diversions to make them time feel like it's going faster. Invest in seek-and-find word games, Sudoku, brochures about the provider, a meet-the-staff bulletin board, Internet access, computer games, fish tanks, an electronic messaging panel with wellness tips, "meet our team" trivia questions, and the like. Inexpensive subscription services can make this very easy.

3. **Underpromise and overdeliver.** Discourage staff from predicting a wait length that is unrealistically short. Encourage staff to proactively shape patients' expectations. Patient satisfaction is tied closely to what the patient has been led to expect about the length of the wait and whether that prediction turns out to be fact or fiction. The moral: In our services, we should be adjusting patient expectations (downward, if necessary) so we can meet or exceed them.

4. **Institute scripts and script rehearsal so that staff members communicate with empathy when informing or updating patients about delays.** Help your team deliver in an authentic way *great* words of apology, explanation, empathy, and appreciation.

5. **Respecting our patients' time and managing our own so we can is not easy.** With open-access scheduling and a multifaceted approach to easing waits in the face of unpreventable delays in care and service, you can win patient appreciation and enhance their experience with your practice.

Health-e-People: E-mail and the Patient Experience

In increasing numbers, patients want to communicate with their physician and their physician's office staff via e-mail. Some physicians complain that e-mail communications are less effective and less satisfying because both patients and physicians miss out on building a personal relationship. Patients see it differently. Some believe that e-mail access is the next best thing to a home visit, and many find their relationship with their physician improving with the informal, personalized communication.

Many solo physicians invite their patients to contact them via e-mail, and some larger practices are instituting e-mail centers that receive e-mails from patients, screen them for issues the center can handle, channel those they can't to the right person, and then follow up to make sure the patient received a response.

Instituting a system to handle patient e-mails is a powerful way to expand access to your practice even if you place limits on what you and your staff can handle via e-mail. Used for the right things, e-mail communication can benefit your patients and your practice. Consider the following benefits:

- **Better access:** E-mail is available to both patient and physician 24/7.
- **No more phone tag with patients:** Patients won't have to wait around for a call-back, and you don't need to try and try again to reach them.
- **Time-saving delegation:** Since some questions can be answered by staff other than you, e-mail reduces unnecessary phone calls on your part, delegating to others who are well-prepared to meet the patient's need.
- **Fewer unnecessary visits and more time for people with complex needs:** When the patient really needs to see you, you can give him or her more time without rushing because you have more time to give and do a better job of building a relationship.
- **Quicker turnaround of test and lab results:** Especially if you use templates, you can save time and satisfy the patient by sending results via e-mail using document management software (e.g., Updox) to attach such information as prescriptions, lab orders, and fact sheets or Web pages, all while sending the information to the patient's electronic health record. However, proceed with caution: You will have to include an automated delivery notice to make sure the patient opened the e-mail with his or her results, and you will also need to make sure your e-mail is secure. These two cautions should not stop you, because options are commercially available that solve these problems.
- **No need to fear Health Insurance Portability and Accountability Act (HIPAA) of 1996 violations:** Online messaging systems are available

so you can implement e-mail communications without violations of HIPAA.

- **Self-documentation:** E-mail can also be self-documenting. You can print and insert e-mails into patient records, or with many electronic medical records, you can copy e-mails to the patient's medical record with the push of a button.

Also to reduce risk, secure servers and digital signature systems are available to protect confidentiality and provide authenticated, secure, and confidential e-mail. At a greater cost, but highly effective, are commercially available systems that allow messages to be triaged based on message type, prescriptions to be auto-faxed, and senders to be automatically notified of successful delivery.

Schedule implications

Consider three service options: face-to-face visits, e-mail, and phone calls. Your schedule can ease up considerably if you shift a portion of your phone calls and face-to-face visits to e-mail contacts. Let's say you see 25 patients a day and talk to another 15 by phone. You would have served a total of 40 patients that day. By using e-mail, you can reduce your face-to-face visits by seeing only the 10 people with complex needs. You can talk to another 5 by phone and interact with another 40 via e-mail. This brings your total for that day to 55. Physicians who use e-mail extensively report numbers like these, showing how e-mail use results in a much more manageable distribution of the physician's time.

Revenue implications

If you have capitated patients, e-mail communication has immediate benefits for both the patient and practice. Your patients can contact you and your team easily, and you can have a more reasonable schedule, seeing fewer patients and being able to spend more time with those with complex needs.

If you have fee-for-service patients, recent changes to CPT codes as of January 1, 2008, include CPT 9444 for e-mail consultation services or "virtual office visits." An e-mail service can be reported only once for the same episode of care in a seven-day period and includes all non-face-to-face communications related to that encounter. You cannot bill separately for follow-up phone calls or orders for drugs, labs, and imaging.

Also, note that the existence of such codes does not ensure payment: Your patients' plans must be willing to reimburse for these codes. Some, such as CIGNA, Aetna, and at least 12 other major insurers are beginning to do so. Each plan determines the physician payment rates and copays for members. Others are instituting reasonable payments for virtual visits because they recognize the cost-effectiveness and positive effect on patient satisfaction. In the absence of insurance payments, some practices are offering e-mail access for an annual subscription fee, while others offer virtual office visits that consumers find so valuable that they pay out of pocket.

The future of e-mail interactions

As financial issues resolve, enhanced access with simple e-mail and Web portals will blossom. In the future, patients and doctors will sit in front of computer screens equipped with video cameras and talk to each other in real-time or leave video messages for each other. The physician will be able to do partial assessments. Voice recognition software will transcribe all communications instantly and shoot them to the patient's electronic medical record, which will be available to both patient and physician. Links will direct the patient to definitions of medical terminology and relevant educational resources. Patients and physicians will answer each other's notes, correcting and elaborating on them, and physicians will send the patient reminders related to wellness and their care plan. Home-based diagnostic technology will send data to clinicians, and patients will send along their questions to the doctor before their visit. When a patient calls the physician, his or her message will be transcribed, converted to e-mail, and sent instantly to the doctor's mobile device. And at any point in the process, communications can be translated into a different language.

Come to terms: Suggested guidelines

If you want to institute or enhance an e-mail communication process with your patients, it's important to establish clear expectations. Outline expectations in a written agreement, discuss them with the patient, and obtain informed consent. Then file or document the signed agreement in the patient's medical record.

FIGURE 3.1   Guidelines for Physician–Patient Agreement on E-mail Use

1. Adjust patient expectations.	• Establish and share with patients a turnaround time for e-mail messages so the patient knows what to expect. The typical time frame is: o Two hours if received before 3 p.m. o By 11 a.m. if received after 3 p.m. the day before • Use automatic reply to relieve patient anxiety about whether the message went through. • When the physician responds, ask for patient confirmation of the receipt of the response, especially for important messages. • Send "out-of-the-office" automatic replies that tell the patient who will respond or whom to call for help.
2. Educate patients about appropriate uses of e-mail.	**Key Message Points** • Here's what's appropriate—for example: o Schedule appointments o Get prescription refills o Ask billing questions o Request a referral o Find out test results o Obtain forms o Get immunization dates o Follow up on medical issues without having to come in o Asking nonurgent medical questions • E-mail is best suited for short communications. For more complex needs, make an office visit. • Don't use e-mail for emergencies. Call 911 or call the office. • Don't e-mail use when the communication is sensitive—for example, when writing about mental health or HIV. • E-mail can't substitute for a physical exam. • If you need an answer before the physician responds to your e-mail, call the office.

FIGURE 3.1 Guidelines for Physician–Patient Agreement on E-mail Use (cont.)

3. Explain what needs to be included in e-mail.	• Pinpoint the subject on the subject line, for example: Referral? Refill? Medical advice? Medication question? • In the body of the message, include the patient name, ID#, and phone number.
4. Explain how privacy will be handled.	**Key message points:** • If you use work e-mail, your employer or possibly a hacker can access it. • All e-mails will be inserted in the patient's medical record. • Members of the physician office staff might handle your message with approval from physician. • Your e-mail address will not be shared or sold for the purpose of marketing. • Clarify circumstances under which the physician might share patient's e-mail with others (e.g., consulting physician).

Figure 3.1 offers some example guidelines that establish common-ground expectations between physician and patient.

Also, assuming you do use e-mail communications, it's worth considering how to refine your writing techniques so that your written words achieve your goals without confusing—or offending—the patient. Consider these tips for e-mail etiquette, or better put, "netiquette."

• Make your e-mail responses gracious and professional. E-mails to patients should feel personal. Call the patient by his or her name, thank him or her for writing, wish the patient well when concluding your message, and suggest that he or she write or call back if in any way concerned or unclear.

- Avoid jargon and write short, simple sentences to be understandable to a wide range of readers in terms of reading levels, familiarity with healthcare lingo, and attention span.

- Don't express anger, criticize, or judge.

- Don't be sarcastic or joke. Despite your positive intent, because the person on the receiving end can't see your face or hear your tone, you risk being misunderstood and offending the patient.

- Use the "blind copy" or BCC function when sending group e-mails so you protect the identity of patients receiving it.

E-mail communication and Web access are revolutionizing many aspects of healthcare. Increasingly, consumers sign on to get and give information, find and evaluate providers, and store personal health information. The enterprising physician and medical practice see this writing on the wall and are finding ways to provide the e-mail access consumers increasingly want.

Phone Finesse

The phone remains the mainstay of communication between patients and physicians. Fortunately, technological solutions are available today that can improve telephone access, efficiency, and customer service. And many insurance companies (e.g., Cigna, Aetna, and at least 12 more major plans) now provide payment for telephone consultations.

As of January 2008, there are new Current Procedural Terminology codes for telephone consultation, thanks to years of teamwork by the American Association of Family Physicians, the American College of Physicians, and the American Academy of Pediatrics. Three codes exist: one for 5–10 minutes, one for 10–20 minutes, and one for 20–30 minutes.

With the possibility of payment and consumers' increasing preference for alternatives to face-to-face visits, telemedicine and improved telephone access are important to provide. Different solutions work for difference practices; the key is to explore technology options and define staff responsibilities that minimize the main frustrations patients experience with physicians' office phone practices.

Patient frustrations with phone access

Patients can become frustrated when they call your practice and:

- Get a busy signal so they have to call back.

- The phone rings endlessly and no one answers.

- Reach a machine message that asks for a name and number and promises a return call that might not happen.

- A staff member answers and puts the patient on hold before he or she can get a word out.

- Hear a recording stating, "All lines are busy. Please hold." Or "We have an unusually high volume of callers right now. Please call back at another time."

- A "call director" system answers, they follow all the directions and push the relevant buttons to reach the department they're calling, and when they are finally connected, they hear a voicemail message.

- Reach a live person from an answering service, but that person knows nothing about the practice and promises in a very impersonal way to convey your message.

- Reach a staff member in the practice, but that person sounds harried or annoyed, or is curt, treating them with a "don't you know I'm busy" attitude.

Five suggestions for improving phone access

1. Check your system's capabilities. First, review your phone system's features and make sure that the system is capable of providing easy access for patients.

2. Define and enforce standards for your answering service team. Recognize that patients view an answering service as part of your practice. Review and adjust the service's scripts so that its scripts align with your vision for your patients' experience with your practice. Insist on a training and orientation process that acquaints their staff with your patient-centered vision, your key people, and services. The agenda should cover the following information:
   - The practice size, services, and staff members
   - The practice's patient-centered philosophy
   - Details about physicians and other key people
   - How to screen calls to trigger appropriate follow-up
   - When to call an ambulance
   - When to contact the doctor on call
   - When to wait until the doctor on call calls in
   - When to call other staff members
   - When to take a message and promise a callback during the practice's regular open hours
   - How to take messages

3. Adjust your staffing. If your staff members who handle phones are inundated with multiple callers and responsibilities (e.g., registering patients), they will not be able to focus and respond to callers with courtesy, grace, appropriate information, patience, and helpfulness. Recognizing this, medical practices are increasingly staffing so that individuals can be dedicated to handling the phones, rather than trying to balance answering the phones with other responsibilities.

4. Institute phone guidelines and scripts for all staff who handle calls. Be sure to address the situations that involve issues of access. How do you want staff to respond to concerned patients so that they reduce, rather than increase, anxiety about access? Also, when callers want to talk with their physician, what promises should the staff make or not make? See Figure 4.1 for a sample script for transferring a call. (Additional guidelines and scripts can be found on the on the accompanying CD-ROM.)

5. Make your phone access practices clear to your patients. Put them in writing, or better yet on a refrigerator magnet for easy access. For most people, the phone is their lifeline to you. When your patients are on the phone, your reputation is on the line.

FIGURE 4.1 Sample Script: Transferring a Call

Instructions	Script
• If the caller needs to reach another office/ staff member, tell the caller which office he or she has reached and offer to transfer the call to the proper office/staff member. Take the time to understand what the caller needs and to figure out who he or she should actually be calling.	• I'm sorry, Mr. Mancini. This is Marge Hoffman in billing. I think you'll want to talk with Harry Hampton to set up an appointment. I'll be glad to transfer your call to Harry. In case you don't reach Harry for some reason, would you like to take down his direct number? Do you have a pencil handy? I'll be glad to wait.
• If you do not have the correct extension at your fingertips, take the time to look it up.	• Harry's number is 456-6666. Would you like me to repeat that for you? Now please hold while I transfer your call, and thank you for calling.
• Be sure to give the caller the correct number for future reference and for use in case the transfer is disconnected.	• [To Harry] Harry, I have Mrs. Hampton on the line, and she'd like to make an appointment.
• When you transfer the call, stay on the line to make sure that you've connected the person with the correct party.	

Continuity of Care

Patients these days want a relationship with their doctors. They want to be recognized and remembered from visit to visit. They also want their care to be continuous and their transitions from one part of our complex health system to another to be seamless; they don't want to fall through cracks. Continuity serves their health outcomes and reduces their anxiety when dealing with matters about their health.

This chapter identifies options related to four types of continuity:

- Treatment from the same doctor every visit
- The seamless visit: Transferring trust between care team members
- Continuity in referrals between you and another provider
- Patient follow-up: Results reporting, adherence monitoring, and disease management

1. Treatment from the same doctor every visit

Patients in every demographic are substantially more satisfied when their appointment is with *their own* primary care physician. People do not want to be bumped to another provider. One benefit of open-access scheduling is its capability of matching patients consistently to their own personal physician.

Whether it is a primary care provider or a specialist, if patients have met a physician before, they expect to be recognized and remembered by the physician. This eases their anxiety and enhances their comfort and overall experience with your practice.

While some providers are naturals at showing personal recognition to the patient at the start of each visit (perhaps they are highly social and have a great memory), others need a triggering process that helps them recognize the patient and convey the "good to see you again" sentiment along with a personal comment or question. Physicians can connect immediately in a personal way by inquiring about something learned from the patient during his or her last visit.

Include a prompt on the patient's chart or electronic medical record that reminds you at the end of a visit to note a personal tidbit you learned about the patient that would be appropriate to mention during his or her next visit. The simplest pieces of information are often the most effective, such as remembering that a patient's son was competing in a tennis championship or that a patient was planning to visit her mother in Pittsburgh.

This kind of personal recognition takes very little effort and eases the patient's anxiety about being "just another patient" to you.

2. The seamless visit: Transferring trust between care team members

With planned teamwork and handoffs among staff members, patients can also experience continuity during a single visit as they move from person to person or service to service. Most patient visits involve a series of handoffs between one person and another—from the receptionist to the nurse or lab tech, or from the nurse or lab tech to the physician. Perhaps you want the patient to return paperwork to the front desk, make payment arrangements or another appointment on his or her way out, or have his or her blood drawn by your nurse or phlebotomist. In each of these situations, the patient's anxiety builds as he or she goes from person to person unless your practice communicates to ensure continuity and understanding about what will happen next and whether they will be well-served by the next person down the line.

At these handoff points, you and your team have opportunities with just a few words to transfer trust and foster confidence in every member of your team. Figure 5.1 illustrates some of the key goals and appropriate wording for handoffs at different stages of the patient care process.

FIGURE 5.1 Key Elements of Transferring Trust

Goals	Examples
Clarify in a patient-centered way the purpose of the handoff.	"Please stop at the front desk and talk to Joan. Before you go, Joan will be glad to set up a convenient appointment for follow-up."
Build the patient's confidence in the service provider on the receiving end of the handoff. Make it clear that, as the patient moves from you to the other person or service, he or she will continue to be in good hands.	"So I'm going to step out and our nurse practitioner, Betsy Wright, will come in to do this procedure with you. She'll tell you exactly what it entails. She's very experienced and very caring. You'll be in good hands with Betsy."
Knowing that anxiety builds at handoff points, invite questions from the patient.	"So before you go, what questions do you have for me? I want you to feel secure about what's next."
If you were on the receiving end of a handoff, express your respect for the caregiver passing the patient along to you.	[To nurse] "Thanks, Helen, for helping Mr. Murphy get ready. [Turning to patient] Mr. Murphy, I can always count on Helen."

Now what's going to happen? Will I know what to do? Will I go the right place and do the right thing? Will the people there be caring? Do they know I'm coming? These are some of the thoughts that are going through patients' minds as they move through your practice. Because anxieties like these escalate at handoff points, it is especially critical to ease the patient's mind by openly expressing your confidence in and respect for the caregiver or service on the other end. This also reinforces coordination of care and teamwork and positions other people in a good light so they will have an easier time earning patients' trust. Also, not only will others on the care team appreciate you for it, but your visible respect will also spark positive word-of-mouth about the team or even create a feeling of family within your practice. Figure 5.2 offers examples of how to execute handoffs that reduce patient anxiety.

FIGURE 5.2 Handoff Dialogue

Situation	Anxiety-reducing dialogue
Handoff to colleague covering for you during your vacation	• "I'll be away when you come in next, but Dr. Marcus will be prepared to see you. Before I go, I'll be sure to talk with her about your needs, so it's very clear. She's a great doctor, and I know you'll be in good hands with her."
Handoff of a complaint	• "I'm so sorry this happened. And I'm glad you brought this to my attention." • "I want to help make it right, Mrs. Jones." • "I would like to talk with our office manager, Sue Johnson, so she can look into this for you. I'll fill Sue in about this, and she'll call you within 24 hours to follow up with you. Okay? And Mrs. Jones, thanks again for speaking up. I want you to have a very good experience with our practice."
Handoff of a child and their companion to the receptionist	• "Okay, Ben, we're all done for today. If you rest up and take your medication, you should start feeling much better in a day or two." • "Ms. Hamilton, I would like to see Ben again in ___ days/weeks to check on ____. On your way out, please stop at the front desk and Suzy will work with you to schedule a convenient appointment." • "But before you go, Ben and Ms. Hamilton, I want to know if either of you has any remaining questions or concerns that I can help you with." • "Please let me know if I've answered your questions or if there are parts that I have not made clear." • "Let me show you two back out to reception where Suzy will be happy to schedule a follow-up appointment for you." • [To receptionist] "Hello Suzy, would you please work with Ms. Hamilton to set up a follow-up appointment for Ben in 10 days?" • "Ben, I hope you'll be feeling better soon! And Ms. Hamilton thanks again for trusting us to care for Ben."

FIGURE 5.2   Handoff Dialogue (cont.)

Handoff to appointment clerk or receptionist (Note: Many patients don't always follow instructions for taking medication or scheduling follow-up appointments. It is much more effective to do a handoff to the appointment clerk to ensure that next appointment is taken care of).	• "Before you go, Helen will help you schedule your follow-up appointment. Let me introduce you to Helen."

When you and your coworkers present yourselves as a connected team of care and service providers who respect and trust one another, you relieve anxieties your patients and their families might go through and build patients' confidence in your entire team. You'll see the results when patients give you high scores on continuity.

3. Continuity in referrals between providers

Patients often find the referral process from your practice to another provider to be confusing and anxiety-provoking. Patients wonder, *Who is this person? Will I be a stranger? Will I have to wait an eternity for an appointment?* When the patient gets what he or she feels is a runaround from the office of the referral provider, the patient becomes frustrated, anxious, and concerned about his or her outcomes. The patient then either waits and worries or calls your office to ask you or your staff to pull strings to get an earlier appointment.

Consider two ways to ease the patient's way to the next provider in the service process and foster the feeling of continuity and seamless care. First, communicate to the patient your trust in the next provider. Help the patient and family to feel secure during the transition, clear about what's happening, and confident about the person on the receiving end. Second, formalize your main referral arrangements. Negotiate written agreements with those to whom you refer that clarify the referral process and enhance continuity for the patient.

Such agreements can help you and your colleagues to be selective in the referrals you make and also consistently thorough in your prereferral information and work-ups. Such agreements can also require specialists receiving the referral to communicate back their findings quickly and thoroughly.

To develop a referral agreement with other providers beyond your practice, you and your team will need to adopt the mindset that you are all part of one system of care. Your goal is to make the system seamless not only within your practice, but also between your practice and others.

Such agreements should also clarify how the referring physician can obtain an immediate consult via cell phone or pager in circumstances that warrant it. To ensure continuity of care for the patient, the referral process also needs to be clear:

- The referring physician can explain to the patient who they will see and within what time frame.
- The process needs to prompt the referring physician to work up and convey needed information in time for the referral date.
- The process should also include parameters that spell out how and by when the specialist will communicate findings to the referring physician.

4. Patient follow-up: Results reporting, patient adherence and support, and proactive disease management

Knowing that patients prefer a long-term relationship with their physicians, managing that relationship requires more than recognition and communication within each visit. For the sake of patient outcomes and patient retention, how you follow up and communicate with patients between visits and over time affects their ability to self-monitor their health, adhere to care plans, and partner with you in adjusting these plans.

Results reporting

Following up on test results may be a procedural headache for your practice, but it is a highly emotional experience for patients and therefore pivotally important. Patients are often unclear about whether they will be notified or have to contact the medical practice for their results. Is no news good news— or does it mean that the practice forgot to follow up? This question causes unnecessary worry and even, at times, avoidable harm. Despite this, less than one-third of physicians have a system that ensures rapid, reliable feedback of results. Many say, "Call me in a week for your results," leaving the responsibility entirely with the patient. Others intend to call patients only with abnormal results, but when these follow-up calls result in telephone tag or fall through the cracks, the patient may wrongly conclude that their results are normal.

Patients want and deserve to be notified of a questionable result. They appreciate calls or e-mails with good news, too. Whatever your patients' results, they expect your practice to follow-up with them responsibly. The data on related causes of malpractice claims substantiate the strength of this expectation among patients.

With manual tracking systems, results management software, and voicemail test result solutions readily available, physicians concerned about the patient experience can easily solve this challenge. The automated solutions make it particularly easy and efficient. For abnormal findings for instance, these systems can:

- Review all chemistry, blood, imaging, and lab results ordered by clinicians and highlight abnormal findings.

- Allow clinicians to see results alongside the patient's previous results, along with a list of the patient's current medications and problems.

- Allow physicians to forward the results with notes to other clinicians involved in the patient's care. Users can also set reminders for repeated testing. Many systems have a fail-safe method of notifying physicians nightly via e-mail if critical results have not been reviewed by other clinicians or the patient.

Support between visits and over time also provides continuity greatly valued by patients, and it increases patient adherence. There are many ways to offer patients support:

- **The checkback call:** Many physicians schedule time daily to make a few follow-up calls to patients. Others delegate the task to a nurse or nurse practitioner. Whether you tell the patient to expect a follow-up call or you surprise them with one, your call makes the patient feel important to you and earns you high marks.

- **The feedback call:** With a feedback call, the physician or designee calls the patient with a test result or other relevant information. Patients resent it when their physician says, "Call me in two weeks for your result." Patients wonder why *they* have to: *Why can't the doctor's office call?* And if the patient forgets, so might the provider, which can easily lead to negative outcomes.

- **E-mail follow-up:** Lately, as more consumers are computer savvy, e-mail is becoming the preferred mode for patient follow-up. Physicians and their staff can send follow-up e-mails at any time of the day or night and the patient will receive those messages whenever he or she signs into his or her e-mail account. E-mail eliminates telephone tag and means much better accessibility between patient and caregiver.

Automated patient follow-up systems and subscription services

Automated follow-up systems facilitate proactive communication with patients. Depending on each patient's preferred method of communication, these systems either automatically send the designated document via e-mail on the due date or direct the user to print and mail the document or call the patient. Many of these systems can be purchased with sets of letters, surveys, and recommended frequencies of communication, or the user can reconfigure a system to reflect another preferred frequency of patient contact. Also, to-do lists can be updated daily and sorted by staff member positions, so each person can work off their own personal to-do list.

Follow-up systems can track patient adherence and progress after visits and can notify patients when they need services, shots, and check-ups. With evidence-based disease management principles built in to drive planned communications, these systems also give people with chronic conditions a new level of confidence that they are managing their disease wisely. You can also generate recall letters for annual physicals and diabetes follow-up visits and produce lists of patients taking specific medications so you can easily identify and reach them if the medication is withdrawn from the market. These capabilities help you more actively manage patients' health and lead to higher levels of patient satisfaction.

Remote patient monitoring

Remote patient monitoring has become a real option thanks to varied patient interfaces, medical devices, and communication links. You can check on the patient and also receive clinical data automatically. Secure bidirectional links make possible a dynamic clinical relationship between the patients and providers. The patient can participate actively by answering drill-down questions related to his or her current condition and risk factors and can receive real-time feedback as well as educational information that help the patient manage his or her chronic illness.

The patient-centered medical home

Another practice model now in an experimental stage holds the promise of reshaping family medicine entirely and easing patients' journey through our complicated, confusing healthcare system. The medical home is designed to provide comprehensive primary care for people regardless of age or medical condition. Patients choose a personal physician, who then engages them in personal goal-setting and manages them throughout all life stages, including preventive, acute, chronic, and end-of-life care. This physician and his or her practice staff provide integrated services, meeting most healthcare needs themselves and arranging care when other professionals are needed. The physician coordinates care across all levels of the healthcare system (e.g., hospitals, subspecialties, home health, and long-term care) and the patient's family and community. The exchange of health information combined with registries and information technology ensures that patients receive appropriate care where and when they need it, in their own language and with sensitivity to their culture.

Although it still needs to be tested and crystallized, this patient-centric model fully engages the patient and offers the hope of providing a better healthcare experience and improved health outcomes.

Above all, patients don't want to get lost or hit roadblocks when navigating our complex and overwhelming healthcare system. Medical practices that design and institute reliable practices for ensuring continuity from person to person and service to service and act on a long-term view of partnership between patient and physician are the ones that win patient favor and loyalty.

The Physician–Patient Relationship

The physician–patient relationship is central to the patient experience. While people commonly blame problems with parking, long wait times, copays, and rude staff members on dissatisfaction with healthcare providers, people rarely change physicians with these problems. The single most powerful determinant of patient satisfaction and patient loyalty in group practices is the physician–patient relationship. In fact, the physician–patient relationship has a greater effect on patient satisfaction and loyalty than all other factors combined.

The fact is that when patients feel a strong connection to their physician, they will tolerate a lot of other frustrations with the practice. Such factors as delays, staff members with attitude problems, trouble getting through on the phone, and inconvenient appointment times are indeed patient dissatisfiers, but they only result in a patient's decision to defect if the physician–patient relationship is disappointing. If the physician–patient relationship is unfavorable, then waiting two months for an appointment to have a 15-minute doctor's visit after a long wait time could push the patient right over the edge.

In the world of medical practice, many factors compete for your attention: relationships with health plans and insurance companies, productivity, market share, hiring and retaining effective office staff, communicating with other physicians, staying abreast of new knowledge and technology, and managing your time and stress, just to name a few. Although all these factors merit energy and attention, medical practices and health plans cannot afford to ignore that the essence of medical care delivery involves interaction between the physician and patient.

Not only does the strength of patients' relationship with their physician have great impact on their decision to stay with or leave the practice, the strength of this relationship also affects a practice's effectiveness and profitability.

Consider these compelling benefits of an exceptional physician–patient relationship:

- **Fewer malpractice claims:** Doctors who can communicate well are less likely to end up in court.
- **Better adherence and better outcomes:** The health of the physician–patient relationship is the best predictor of whether the patient will adhere to his or her physician's instructions and advice. And this adherence leads to more positive health outcomes.
- **Greater patient satisfaction and retention:** The interaction between physician and patient is the most powerful determinant of patient satisfaction in group practice settings. It is also has the greatest influence on patient loyalty.

- **Enhanced job satisfaction:** Your work is more satisfying and less stressful. Research shows that if you build patient-centered relationships, you are less likely to burn out and more likely to reap mental rewards from your work.

Consider this: In a review of 14 studies of physician–patient communication, researchers found that factors positively related to patient outcomes included reassurance, empathy and support, patient-centered questioning techniques, perceived encounter length, the quality of explanations given, the physician's friendliness and courtesy, orienting the patient as the visit progresses, and summarizing and clarifying findings and recommendations.[1] Notice a trend? The elements of the physician–patient relationship with the greatest impact on patient satisfaction and retention all involve communication.

This section provides a refresher on and specific tools related to salient aspects of the physician–patient relationship. By sharpening your use of these skills and tools, you will reap even more of their multiple benefits.

The story of the master swordsmen

In Japan, master swordsmen endure a complicated training regimen consisting of many moves and subskills. The swordsmen study these skills in depth, one skill at a time. Those who are natural swordsmen often have an awkward time, noting that they perform worse when focusing on one skill at a time. But they persist in completing the exercises.

Once they have mastered the skills individually, they make a trek to a mountaintop to meditate. During their meditation, they deliberately let go of what they learned. They forget it. And lo and behold, after returning from their trek, they find that the specific skills that they learned in a tedious fashion had become integrated and natural and are now automatic for them. They rarely give another thought to a single skill.

If you choose to experiment with the skills described in this section, you too might find yourself feeling self-conscious and awkward when focusing intently on one skill at a time. But soon, they will become integrated into your natural style and enable you to consistently impress your patients with your competence and caring.

 On the accompanying CD-ROM you'll find a variety of tools related to the material in Section II, including tools to improve:

- Greetings
- Handoffs
- Goodbyes
- Presence
- Acknowledging feelings
- Expressing caring nonverbally
- Explaining positive intent

- Offering the blameless apology
- Giving the gift of positive regard
- Using the caring broken record

Endnotes

1. Beck RS, Daughtridge R, Sloane PD. Physician-patient communication: A systematic review. *J American Board of Family Practice.* 2002 Jan–Feb;15(1):25–38.

Effective Visit Openings and Closings

The opening of the visit creates the patient's first impression and affects patient trust and how the visit proceeds from that moment on. How you end the visit then creates the patient's last *and lasting* impression as he or she leaves and reflects on the experience.

This chapter describes how you can invest in great openings and closings so your patients feel connected to you, cared about, and clear about the agenda as the visit proceeds and ends.

Invest in openings

There are four components of an effective patient-visit opening:

1. The first hello
2. Greeting the patient by name
3. Connecting to the person, not the condition
4. Setting the agenda and expectations

1. The first hello

Starting with the first hello, it takes six seconds to create a first impression. If the first impression you make is positive, you establish rapport quickly, reduce the patient's anxiety, and establish a climate of goodwill and cooperation for the visit.

How to establish quick rapport

- Knock before you enter the exam room.

- Give a warm welcome. Make eye contact and smile.

- Immediately call the patient by his or her name.

- Introduce yourself to the patient (and companion, if present) if you haven't met before.

- Pay undivided attention so the patient feels important immediately.

- Apologize if the patient has been kept waiting.

- If you have met the patient before, ask about something personal that you learned during your last contact with them (e.g., "You were on your way to see your son's championship game last time. Did he win?"). Make this easier for yourself by noting some personal info in the patient's chart for use next time.

- Encourage patients to communicate so they can get the help they came for.

- Relate to the patient in a personal way before you get to the business at hand.

---

2. Greeting the patient by name

When it comes to using names, remember two keys: People love hearing their name, so use it often, and always use their *preferred* name. People want to be called what they want to be called.

Remember the following guidelines when using a patient's name:

- Call the patient by first and last name initially and quickly find out what he or she prefers to be called.
- If patients prefer to be called by their first name, use it and thank them, since this is a privilege they're granting you.
- Use the preferred name immediately so you'll remember it.
- Use the preferred name again and again thereafter.

And beware. Certain nicknames are high-risk. Avoid names like *honey, sweetheart, dear, granny, mom, sonny,* etc. Although nicknames may be well-intentioned and some people might not mind them, they are known to breed resentment in the majority of patients and their families. Call people by name instead.

If you're thinking we're being too restrictive or that your patients wouldn't react badly to a nickname consider this: Imagine you're sick with a disease. There are two drugs that cure the disease, drug A and drug B. Both cure the disease, but drug B sometimes has negative side effects. Which drug would you want? Drug A, of course. Why risk negative side effects? Calling patients "honey" and "sweetheart" is like using drug B and risking an adverse reaction.

To make your greeting even more effective, build into it elements that will ease the patient's anxieties. Note in Figure 6.1 how the physician's greeting eases anxiety specific to the circumstances of the patient–physician interaction.

FIGURE 6.1 Greetings Tailored to Special Circumstances

Situation	Likely patient anxieties	Anxiety-reducing greeting
A colleague is away. You are seeing this colleague's patient.	• Will this doctor be nice? • Will my doctor know what's happening with me?	"Hello, Mr. Samson. I'm Dr. [Colleague]. I'm sorry Dr. [YourDoctor] isn't available today, but I'll be glad to help you. And I'll be sure to let Dr. [YourDoctor] know all about your visit. So tell me: What brings you here today?"
You are a specialist. A primary care physician referred his patient to you.	• Will this doctor be nice? • Will this doctor care about me? • Will this doctor and my doctor communicate so one hand knows what the other hand is doing?	"Hello, Mr. Granger. It's nice to meet you. I'm Dr. Miller. I understand Dr. [YourDoctor] referred you to me, and I'll be glad to help. And after our visit, I'll be sure to communicate with Dr. [YourDoctor] about our visit."
You're called to do a consult with a hospital patient.	• Now who's this? This isn't my doctor! • Does my doctor know about this? • Who's making the final decisions?	"Hello, Mr. Samson. It's very nice to meet you. I'm Dr. Consult, and Dr. [YourDoctor] asked me to see you about your ___. After my visit with you, I'll be sure to connect with Dr. [YourDoctor] and let him know all about it, since he oversees your care."

FIGURE 6.1 Greetings Tailored to Special Circumstances (cont.)

A patient's family member arranges to talk with you about his or her loved one.	Will this doctor care? Will this doctor really hear my concerns?	"Hello, Mrs. Garver. It's nice to meet you. It's great that your mother has your support. Now, how can I help you?"
You pass people in hallways and other public areas while walking around the facility.	Who are all these people? This place is a maze. Will I find where I'm supposed to be? I'm out of my element here.	• Wear your name badge where others can easily see it. • Make eye contact, smile, and say hello as you pass. • Hold doors and yield to patients and visitors. • If someone looks lost, offer help.
You take a phone call.	Who is this? Will this busy doctor concentrate on me?	• Take a breath before answering. • Smile (people can hear it in your voice). • Identify yourself (and if unknown to the patient, your role.

3. Connecting to the person, not the condition

To establish rapport quickly after the initial greeting, adopt a routine that enables patients and family members to immediately feel your interest in them as individuals—before you focus on the patient's complaint or need.

Many physicians are concerned that they don't have time to establish a rapport with patients. Yet many studies show that it takes skillful physicians less than a minute to obtain a quick profile of the patient as a person.

Consider the following tactics:

- If it is the patient's first visit, get to know him or her right away and begin earning trust by asking a few personal questions about work, family, personal interests, and other similar topics.
- Another option with a new patient: Begin addressing the biomedical facts first, but then in the process make room for personal questions.
- For return patients, ask for an interim report. Show that you remember them from the previous visit.
- Make notes on the patient's chart so you can cue yourself to check in from visit to visit.
- Thank the person for sharing with you.

4. Setting the agenda and expectations

Setting the agenda for the visit in partnership with the patient helps both you and the patient manage time during the visit. The more thoroughly you do this, the fewer surprises you'll have at the end of the visit, when the patient says, "And doctor, one more thing . . ." Or, "Doctor, by the way . . ."

Follow these four steps to set the visit agenda:

1. Listen. Find out the patient's agenda and clarify his or her expectations to avoid last-minute add-ons by asking, "What else?" before proceeding.
2. Add your items to the list of concerns.
3. Negotiate the agenda if necessary. If you're unsure if the patient's entire agenda can be accomplished in this visit, explain why and establish a timeline for what can be accomplished during this visit and what should wait until later.
4. Foreshadow. Explicitly explain what the patient can expect during each stage of the visit.

Contrary to common opinion, taking a couple of minutes to allow patients to state all of their concerns up front without interruption does not add to the length of the interview. Also, getting on the same wavelength as the patient right from the start will make it easier for you to anticipate and respond to the patient's concerns as the visit proceeds.

Invest in closings

The last few minutes of the patient's visit not only influence his or her satisfaction with the care provided, but they also influence patient adherence to physician instructions and the outcomes the patient will experience as a result.

Patients report the following closing approaches to be ineffective at best or insulting at worst:

- *"Is there anything else?"* This is better when asked early in the visit. Toward the end of the meeting, if the patient brings up something new, it tends to frustrate the physician and he or she is likely to rush, leaving the patient with a feeling of ill will.

- *No goodbye at all.* Suddenly the physician disappears and another staff member arrives and closes the interaction.

- *"I have to go."* Patients say this feels dismissive. The feeling of being rushed out can be insulting.

- *"Sit here and someone will be with you."* This might be appropriate to the upcoming tasks, but there is no "goodbye" in it. It fails to produce closure between the physician and patient for that visit.

- *"I have other patients to take care of."* Patients know this fact and find this line patronizing and discounting. It's much better to say, "We'll need to end now since other patients are waiting. So I can give the other concerns you just raised the time they deserve, would you like to make another appointment?"

- *"Good luck."* Imagine needing a knee replacement and your surgeon says to you the day before surgery, "Good luck." This would not ease your mind. Although saying "good luck" certainly stems from goodwill, in healthcare, the words "good luck" tend to increase patient anxiety. Patients don't want to think about the possibility that they need luck to have a positive outcome. It's much better to say, *"I hope all goes well for you."*

- *"Don't worry about your mother. She'll be fine."* When said to a family member, this feels belittling and discounts the family member's very real concern. It's better to show appreciation of this family member's care and dedication.

- *"We'll need to end now. I have to go pick up my kids."* This statement is about the physician, not the patient. A great goodbye ends with a line that is patient-centered. It's fine to say "I'll be leaving now, because I have to pick up my kids" as long as you go on to say, "Is there anything more I can do for you before I go?" Then, "Goodbye, Mrs. Smith. Good to see you."

The most effective strategies for wrapping up a medical visit involve shifting the patient's focus to the future, finalizing and reviewing plans, checking that the patient understands his or her plan of care, and saying goodbye. Figures 6.2 and 6.3 contain tips for managing closings as well as suggested language to use.

FIGURE 6.2   Closings that Work

Steps	Words that work
Alert the patient that the visit is ending: • Smile, make eye contact • Address the patient again by name • Say closing words that help prepare the patient for the end of the visit	• "Mr. Johnson, we have just a few minutes left today. Is there one more question I can answer for you before we end?" • "So Ben, we're nearing the end of your visit . . . I'm happy to address one more question before we end."
Review what occurred, the plan for the patient, and any next steps. Be sure to go over the medication or treatment plan and when you next want to see the patient. Some physicians do this at the end of the visit regarding all of the patient's concerns. Others do mini-summaries, providing closure after the discussion of each of the patient's concerns.	"So as we wrap up today, let's make sure we're on the same page. Here's what I learned, and here's the plan we've agreed on. We'll take a look at your blood results in two weeks to make sure you're moving in the right direction. I'd like to see you in six weeks. After you leave, your part will involve . . ."
Check the patient's understanding and acceptance.	• "So what's your understanding of what you need to do next? I want to be sure I've been clear and thorough." • "And how are you feeling about proceeding that way?"
Be sure the patient knows what to expect and what to do if the condition gets better or worse. Clarify how the patient can contact you (or others) if needed.	• "I expect you to start feeling better by . . ." • "If your symptoms are getting better, then I want you to . . ." • "Mr. Jones, if any of your symptoms worsen or you have concerns, please call me and let me know. The best way to reach me is . . ."

FIGURE 6.2   Closings that Work (cont.)

If you can honestly do so, offer reassurance.	• "I think you're going to feel better fast by following our plan." • "If this medication doesn't work for you, we can talk again and try alternatives."
Wrap up the encounter with caring comments. Connect personally.	• "I really want that cough to subside so you can get some peace." • "I hope you feel great in time for your daughter's big event!" • "Thanks for coming in (or choosing our practice). It's always good to see you." • "I hope you feel better fast. And please send my regards to Harriet and the kids."

FIGURE 6.3   Tips for Problematic Closings

Special circumstance	Tips	Words That Work
When the patient has sprung new issues on you and you are out of time	Acknowledge the importance of the new items. If you believe the issue is not urgent and can wait, explain that you want to address it when you can give it your full attention. If the issue can't wait, deal with it or find someone who can. And let it serve as a reminder to you that it saves time to urge the patient to express his or her entire agenda early on.	"I'm glad you brought this to my attention. To deal with it adequately, I'll need more time to talk with you. I'd like to schedule another appointment so I can give this the time it deserves. How does that sound?"
When you need to leave the room before completing the visit (e.g., to go for meds, scrips, or instruction sheets)	When you return, sit down. This might seem counterintuitive since you are trying to end the visit, but research has shown that the non-verbal act of sitting down creates positive perceptions on the part of the patient. Also, if you sit down, you can then stand up at a later point to signal the need to wrap-up.	"One more thing . . . I'm going to get those samples for you. When I come back, we'll talk about how to take the medication, and then we'll be through for today."
When you're saying goodbye to a coworker (Mark) to whom you've just handed off your patient (Mrs. Harris)	Don't let your coworker feel invisible to you. Acknowledge your coworker and complement him or her in front of the patient.	"Is there anything else you need from me on my end, Mark? Okay then, thanks so much for taking care of Mrs. Harris. Mrs. Harris, you're in good hands with Mark."

FIGURE 6.3 Tips for Problematic Closings (cont.)

| When you're saying goodbye to a patient on the phone | Don't let the conversation fizzle. Endings like "okay," "bye," "uh huh," or not saying goodbye at all tend to leave patients feeling dismissed and discounted. End on a positive note. Summarize what you're going to do for the caller and by when. Invite questions, use the caller's name, thank them, and add on a few caring words. Let the caller hang up first. You'll know they are finished and won't risk having the caller feel as though you cut the call short. | • "Okay Mrs. Jones, I'll find out that info and get back to you by tomorrow evening."
• "Mrs. Jones, what else can I do for you today?" |

•

Closings have a disproportionately large effect on the patient experience. As the patient leaves, he or she remembers best those precious last few minutes with you. The more you can do early in the visit to prevent interrupted, rushed, or dissatisfying closings, the easier the closing will be for you and the better the impression you'll make on the patient. Most crucial, by perfecting your closing communication, you make the most of this last opportunity to ease the patient's anxiety and leave the patient with a positive last impression of you and your practice.

The Power of Presence

There is one powerful approach above all others that positively influences patient perceptions of "the time spent with the physician"—an approach that doesn't require more time on your part. In fact it often requires less.

Picture this: The physician enters the exam room several minutes late, writes notes furiously, and turns away while the patient is talking. The patient perceives the physician as impatient and unplugged. Over several encounters, the patient interprets such nonverbal behavior as a message that his or her visit is unimportant, despite many spoken assurances to the contrary.

Whether patients perceive you as "all there" significantly impacts their perception of the quality of their experience with you. Physicians need to express "respectful attention" nonverbally, and this is the most powerful way to build a relationship with patients. It's not a matter of paying more attention to patients; it's a matter of paying better attention to patients.

The Consumer Assessment of Healthcare Providers and Systems (CAHPS) and other patient satisfaction surveys ask patients to rate "the time spent with the physician." But who has more time to give?

Consider this established fact: If two physicians each spend 10 minutes with a patient and one of those physicians appears friendly and helpful and the other curt and rushed with his hand on the doorknob, the patient actually perceives the caring physician as having spent more time. The *quality* of the time spent has more to do with perception of time than does the *quantity* of time spent.

Improving quality, reducing quantity

Patients sense when you are distracted. When you look down or away, when you nod or say "uh huh" with a vacant stare, when you lose eye contact while jotting notes on a chart or computer, when you turn away while the patient is talking, when you look at your watch while nodding, and when you answer your cell phone in mid-conversation, the patient concludes that your mind and heart are elsewhere. Most patients then have a large internal reaction, feeling unimportant and becoming anxious about getting the help they need.

The one skill most powerful in creating positive perceptions of "time spent with the physician" is the skill of "presence" or "mindfulness."

> ### Presence: A working definition
> 1. The state of being consciously and compassionately in the present moment with another. Giving the patient your undivided attention. Fully focusing on the patient in the here and now—body and mind, heart and soul.
> 2. Presence thrives in an attitude of loving kindness and generosity, not judgment or impatience.

Physicians who have improved their presence in a determined fashion have found that it actually saves them time. Because their concentration is better, the patient is more relaxed and trusting, and the visit goes more smoothly. More good news: These physicians found that it helps tune them in to their caring mission, making the experience of being a physician more gratifying.

Without using words, a physician with presence communicates to the patient, "You are not an item on my to-do list. You, uniquely you, matter to me. And I want to know you and your concerns so I can support your health."

Developing the mental discipline

Being present with another person is a *practice*. It takes ongoing consciousness and commitment to grow it. Consider the following tips:

- Take a deep breath. Bring your attention to the present moment and the person at hand.

- Move to the person's level. Sit when they're sitting.
- Shift to a posture of presence. Place your legs evenly on the floor. Open your palms. Relax your belly. Smile and sustain eye contact.
- Face the person fully.
- Don't think about what you're going to do next.
- When you sense yourself becoming distracted, cue yourself silently to refocus on the person. Take a deep breath and bring your attention to the present moment. Put the person in the foreground of your mind.
- If you need to divert your attention, instead of just doing it, *explain while maintaining presence.*
- If you need to end the conversation, instead of giving subtle cues that make you seem absent, *say it directly and kindly while remaining present.*

Also beware of the behaviors that patients perceive as inattentive, or possibly disrespectful, on your part:

- Being silent or unresponsive
- Turning your back without apologizing and explaining (or even slightly turning away)
- Walking away with no explanation or goodbye
- Acting tired, bored, or distracted
- Looking at your watch
- Muttering
- Interrupting

Be aware of your behavior, and work to hone the skill of being present any-time and anywhere—with patients and coworkers and with your family and friends.

Presence on the phone

The power of presence also applies to the important interactions you have with patients on the phone. Many of the same tactics that can improve presence face to face also work over the phone. Stop doing other things and give the patient your full attention, for example. Pay attention to posture—sit up, take a deep breath, and smile (even though the patient can't see you). Concentrate on tuning in, and this will help you automatically tune out other distractions. If someone interrupts, smile at the person and gesture to please wait. If you must answer another call or respond to someone else, explain that to your caller and thank the person for understanding. Also avoid putting the patient on speakerphone—the caller hears everything.

How is your presence? Take a look by addressing the questions in Figure 7.1.

When you are present, patients perceive your focus and caring. This helps them feel less anxious, more trusting, and grateful—and they are more likely to adhere to your advice. Best of all, presence doesn't take more time. It improves the quality of time spent, giving you maximum information because of your undivided attention and making patients feel like you've spent the right amount of time with them.

FIGURE 7.1   Presence Self-Check

Am I present to my patients and families? Do I . . .	Never	Sometimes	Most of the time	Always
1. Shift to a posture of "presence" (place my legs evenly on floor, open my palms, relax my stomach)?				
2. Face the person I'm talking with so I can see the color of the person's eyes on his or her level?				
3. Take a deep breath and bring my attention to the present moment?				
4. Notice my stray thoughts, acknowledge them, and let them go, bringing the person at hand back into the foreground of my mind?				
5. Cue myself silently when I sense myself becoming distracted to refocus on the person in the present moment (telling myself, "Be here now; connect")?				
6. Keep track of time without repeatedly looking at my watch?				
7. Make sure to make eye contact (e.g., not look at the computer screen) when I'm asking questions or listening?				
8. If I need to divert my attention, instead of just doing it, I explain while maintaining presence?				
9. End a conversation by saying directly and nicely that I need to do so, all while remaining present?				

Presence and the computer

Two technological developments have had an enormous impact on physician communication and patient satisfaction: the computer and the personal digital assistant (PDA). Researchers have demonstrated that computer use during consultations has an adverse effect on the quality of interpersonal communication and a consequent negative affect on patient satisfaction.[1] When you have an electronic medical record and in-room computer, how do you avoid giving the patient the impression that you are unplugged from them when you're plugged into the computer?

Second, in this age of instant communication and e-mail, how do you cater to patients who want e-mail communication with you and your team without losing time?

The good news is that both can be accomplished without compromises.

The myth of multitasking

These days, multitasking is considered to be a job (and life) requirement. Yet research shows that multitasking is a myth: People cannot actually do two things at once. What we call "multitasking" would be better termed as "rapid shifting," or quickly alternating from one thing to another. And some people are better at making those rapid shifts than others.

Consider that multitasking:

- Is inefficient. Every time you shift your attention, you lose a bit of time during the transition.

- Is perceived by patients and families as inattentive, if not insulting.

- Causes you to miss important information. When you take notes while a patient is talking, you might miss nonverbal cues and absorb less fully what the patient is saying. Not only can this affect your effectiveness, it can also make it necessary to ask more questions and spend more time getting the information you missed.

So to return to the earlier question: When you have a patient in the room and also expect or need to enter or access information via computer, how can you tune in to the computer without giving patients the impression that you are tuning out on them?

It helps to become so familiar with typing and using the computer that it requires minimal attention. This makes it easier to keep the patient in the foreground while accessing on-screen information and taking notes in the background. Still, clinicians are rarely able to multitask at this level and thus cannot concentrate on the patient and computer at the same time.

The best practice regarding computer use is to alternate your attention to the patient and to the computer, making clear when you are switching from one to the other. For instance, listen intently to the patient and then say, "Give me a moment. I want to make a note of that." Then turn to the computer and enter the information. Don't try to do both at the same time.

FIGURE 7.2 Staying Connected to Both the Person and the Computer

Connect Personally Up front	Find Out the Patient's Perspectives	Show Empathy
• Log onto the computer and look up patient's chart before he or she enters the room. Brief yourself on historical info and personal notes about the patient/family. • Tell the patient about the computer and how your use of it will benefit you and him or her. • Take a look at relevant intake and nursing notes. Review past results. • CONNECT PERSONALLY. Mention something non-medical about the person, his or her past history, or reason for being here. • Reassure the patient about confidentiality. • Ask open-ended questions to learn about the patient and his or her needs and preferences.	• Place the screen so you can see both the patient AND screen. • Ask the patient for his or her thoughts and ideas. • Enter subjective data. • Invite patient/family reactions and thoughts. • Ask the patient/family to verify info. • Ask family members' ideas too. • Find out the patient's goal today. • Explain what you're doing as you enter information into the computer. • Welcome the patient to view the screen. • Engage the patient and his or her significant other in decisions.	• Note body cues and tone of voice. • Reflect back the feeling you think you're hearing. Check out your understanding. • Compliment your patient on what he or she is already doing to deal with the need or concern. • Turn your whole self toward the patient and maintain eye contact. • Stay tuned in; show it (expression, touch). Stay connected to the patient and be present. • Express empathy in your words and nonverbal behavior. • Be conscious of yourself and the focus of your attention.

Staying present to patients when you are using a computer, PDA, or chart has a positive impact on four of the CAHPS survey questions about patient perceptions of their physicians:

1. **Did the physician listen carefully to you?** If you are focusing on the computer while the patient is talking, the patient's perception is that you are not really listening. By clearly transitioning from the person to the computer and back and being very attentive when listening to the patient, even if you then shift to look at the computer, the patient is more satisfied.

2. **Did the physician explain things so you could understand?** By explaining why you are using the computer and how it will help care for the patient, patients feel clearer and more tolerant of your use during office visits.

3. **Did the physician show respect for what you had to say?** If you are not giving the patient your full attention when they are talking, this too is interpreted as a sign of lack of interest on your part.

4. **Did the physician spend enough time with you?** When physicians remain present to the patient when communicating, the patient perceives the time the physician spent with them as longer than an objectively longer visit in which the physician's attention appeared scattered.

Use the checklist in Figure 7.3 to assess your current habits when interacting with both a computer and a patient.

FIGURE 7.3   Computer Communication Self-Check

When interacting with both a computer and a child or parent, do I . . .	Always	Most of the time	Sometimes	Never
1. Connect with the people first, before working at the computer?				
2. Explain the computer in a way that reduces anxiety?				
3. Focus my eyes and turn my full body toward the person while speaking or listening (not toward the computer or over my shoulder)?				
4. Make a clear transition between listening and attending to computer (e.g., saying, "Let me take a minute to make some notes here, please")?				
5. Give patient/customer choices/ options?				
6. Assure confidentiality				
7. Maintain a positive demeanor and thank my customer?				

When using a computer with the patient in the room, presence, not multitasking, is the best practice. When you alternate clearly between giving full attention to the patient and then, with an explanation, giving full attention to the computer, you benefit from the computer's benefits without negatively impacting the patient experience.

Endnotes

1. Booth N, Robinson P, Kohannejad, J. *Inform Primary Care.* 20041–12(2):75–83(2004).

8

Engaging the Patient to Improve Outcomes

While patients depend on you for guidance, information, answers, options, and suggestions, many want to be involved in their own diagnosis, treatment, and planning process. Even those who may not choose to be involved can benefit if you encourage them to be partners in their own care.

The Consumer Assessment of Healthcare Providers and Systems (CAHPS) survey includes several items that reveal behaviors on the part of the physician that are important to patient involvement and engagement and affect the quality of patient involvement and outcomes.

FIGURE 8.1   CAHPS Survey Questions

CAHPS question: Did the physician . . .	Communication skills
Listen carefully to you?	When you ask effective open-ended questions, patients and their companions feel your openness to and interest in them and their perspective.
Show respect for what you have to say?	When you invite questions in an open way, listen well, and check your understanding, patients feel your respect. This encourages their participation in their own care.
Spend enough time with you?	• When you check your understanding and theirs, the communication feels thorough and complete, making the time spent feel adequate at the very least. The patient is less likely to feel shortchanged or rushed. • When you ask open-ended questions and listen to the answers, patients feel heard. Because they have expressed their needs and you have listened, they expect that you are better able to meet their needs. They conclude that the visit was successful—that together you have accomplished the purpose of their visit.
Explain things so you could understand?	By providing "care-full" explanations, checking the patient's understanding, and clarifying as needed, the patient is certain to respect your efforts to be clear and understandable.

Patient engagement is challenging because the physician–patient relationship is lopsided. The patient is the expert on his or her experience—what he or she is thinking, feeling, assuming, and doing about what ails him or her. The physician is the expert on the biomedical aspects—the symptoms, research, diagnosis, options, and prognosis. If the physician does an ineffective job of eliciting the knowledge the patient uniquely holds, the physician has an incomplete picture of what's happening for the patient and will be less able to provide quality care. Also, if the physician fails to get through to the patient, the patient's grasp of information, consideration of options, ownership of decisions, and adherence to plans will be hampered.

Exchanging information and establishing mutual understanding are not easy. Several barriers stand in the way:

- Patients tend to be anxious and feel unsophisticated compared to the highly-trained physician.
- Patients are nervous at the doctor's office, making it hard to concentrate.
- Patients come with their own preconceived ideas about their health, which can make it hard to hear and absorb the physician's ideas.
- Language and cultural differences can make communication all the more difficult.
- Physicians have little time and an eagerness to finish can truncate important discussion and explanations.

Forming a partnership

Despite these barriers, truly patient-centered practices respect and build on information and understanding. They recognize that effective healthcare requires a partnership with the patient—a partnership characterized by a mutual exchange of information, discussion of options, shared decision-making, and responsibility for adherence to wellness and care plans.

Although innovative practices like this are powerful, your everyday communication practices (i.e., how you question, listen, explain and check understanding) are most critical to patient satisfaction and positive outcomes.

Six ways to elicit information

Not only patient satisfaction, but also the efficiency and effectiveness of a visit, depend on your ability to get your patient to open up. Patients need to describe their activities and symptoms and express their feelings, concerns, expectations, ideas, and preferences to relieve their own anxiety about the visit and their presenting need. They also need to talk to provide you with the information you need to meet their needs. Here's a quick refresher on six ways to elicit the patient's experience, perspective, and needs.

1. Encourage patients to prepare

Patients often become anxious when going to see a doctor. This anxiety can make it hard for the patient to think straight and remember his or her concerns and questions. This then makes it hard to set the agenda for the visit and uncover what might be a multifaceted picture of what's going on. The patient's agenda and questions come out in dribs and drabs during the visit. The infamous "doorknob moment"—when a patient suddenly remembers "one more thing" after you think the visit is over—plays havoc with your time and schedule.

To help avoid that the doorknob moment, institute a script for your appointment clerk to use after scheduling a visit for the patient—for instance, "I know Dr. Jones will want to address your concerns and questions when you come. May I suggest that you jot down your symptoms and any concerns and questions and bring that list to show the doctor when you come?"

Not only can patient question lists help you get to the heart of the matter quickly, but patients will also be impressed with your determination to address their concerns. You can also be more efficient because you have the information you need that will enable you and the patient to negotiate a manageable agenda for the visit.

When the patient arrives for his or her visit, if the patient will need to wait even five minutes before seeing the doctor, offer the patient a pad and pencil or a form to complete for jotting down questions and concerns.

Sample patient preparation form

Dear patient,

Please take a few moments to jot down all of your concerns and questions so you and your doctor can make the best use of the time you have together today.

1. What has happened recently that you think the doctor should know about? What do you want to be sure to inform the doctor about?
2. What symptoms or concerns do you want to discuss with your doctor?
3. What questions do you have for your doctor? (Don't hold back. There is no such thing as a bad question!)
4. What's most important to discuss today?

Please take this list into the exam room with you. Thank you.

By prompting patients to formulate their questions and concerns in advance, you make it easier to provide the needed care. No more fishing for their main concerns or giving short shrift to concerns revealed at the end of the visit.

2. Delegate history-taking to the patient

Software is available that allows patients to enter their information from home, in writing at your office, or at a terminal you can provide in a private cubicle. This practice saves you time and provides you with more complete information because patients take time to think about their symptoms, their reasons for scheduling an appointment with you, and their questions.

As the personal health record becomes an increasingly viable option, some patients will be much more involved in maintaining an accurate medical history record.

3. Ask open-ended questions

When you want to learn about the patient's experience and perspective, closed-ended questions—which can be answered with yes or no—don't work: They lead to short answers and fail to help the patient open up. And many patients perceive them as insincere invitations to talk. They feel rushed or brushed off. You then miss valuable information that would influence your thinking and the care you provide.

In contrast, open-ended questions help patients express themselves. These cannot be answered with one word, nor can the patient guess "the right answer." To answer open-ended questions, the patient needs to think and then share his or her ideas. Figure 8.2 includes examples of both types of questions.

FIGURE 8.2 Closed- and Open-Ended Questions

Closed-ended	Open-ended
Are you okay?	How are you feeling? What feels unfinished or unclear for you at this point?
Is there anything else you want to know?	What else do you want to know about this before going?
You're making terrific progress, don't you think?	What progress, if any, do you think you're making?
Is your stomach better?	How is your stomach feeling today?
Do you want me to talk to your mom about this?	What about this would you want me to discuss with your mom?
Do you understand?	So what's your understanding of what you'll need to do?
To a patient's family member: • Do you understand what to do for your mother? • Do you have any questions before you go?	To a patient's family member: • How do you see your role with your mother this next week? • What questions do you have before you go?

Consider too the special power of the question, "What else?"—as in, "What else do you want to discuss today?" At the beginning of a medical interview, you can extract the patient's entire agenda by asking this question several times. Doing so can reduce the occurrence of, and therefore the frustration caused by, doorknob moments after you think the visit is over.

4. Check your understanding

After successfully encouraging patients to express themselves, you can proceed to build their trust in you by showing them that you heard what they said.

By paraphrasing the content of patients' words and reflecting back the feelings you think they're having, you eliminate miscommunications and show your patients you are listening and care enough to get it right.

Example:

Patient: The pain starts on the right side.

Doctor: Over on the right side of your chest?

Patient: Yes, and it is a really sharp pain.

Doctor: Not an ache, but more of a sharp pain?

Beyond paraphrasing, there is even greater value in checking your read on the patient's feelings and concerns. Patients want to feel understood. When you reflect back to them the feelings you think they're projecting, they interpret this as caring on your part, and they appreciate you for it.

Checking your understanding of the patient's feelings allows you to act on a full picture of what's happening with this patient.

5. Invite patient questions and mean it

Since many patients expect to be rushed, they especially appreciate the physician who invites their questions in a genuine way. They perceive this respect as an invitation to partner in their own care. They also absorb what the physician is saying because he or she provides information in the patient's terms in a just-in-time fashion.

Consider these examples:

- "We're nearing the end of your visit. Before you go, I want to make sure you feel clear and confident about how to follow up. Do you have any questions about anything we've discussed?"

- "Let's check, just to be sure I've been clear: What other questions do you have about medication, rest, follow-up care, what you can eat, etc.?"

- "I want you to know how to reach me [one of us] if you have questions after you leave."

6. Give patients a chance to think and explain

After you encourage the patient to talk, give him or her a chance to think and explain. Did you know that physicians typically wait only 18 seconds after a patient begins describing his or her chief complaint before interrupting and redirecting the discussion? Such "premature redirection" makes it more likely that the patient will suddenly expand the agenda at the end of the visit. It also reflects a missed opportunity to gather important data. Maintain gentle eye contact, use silence, and pause after you've asked the patient a question.

Four ways to communicate knowledge and suggestions effectively

Not only must you understand the patient, but the patient must clearly understand you to have an effective visit. If you aren't clearly communicating information to the patient, he or she may misinterpret your diagnosis or treatment advice. Consider these four pieces of advice to improve patient–physician communication.

1. Talk plainly

Have you ever thought after talking to someone, "He talked and talked, but I have no idea what he said!" It's not an uncommon patient complaint. Try your best to avoid jargon and acronyms and use the patient's own words.

To avoid frustrating the patient and to lay the groundwork for adherence to your suggestions, the patient has to understand you. PRN, CXR, DNR, PO, HMO, PE, AAA, CABG, GSW, INR, lap chole . . . and of course the list goes on. Although medical jargon is great shorthand for providers communicating with one another, it makes laypeople feel insecure and anxious and interferes with their comprehension of what's going on. Patients also resent a physician's use of acronyms and jargon because they feel that he or she should know better than to use words that patients don't understand.

Patients also complain when their physicians make them feel inferior by speaking with long or obscure words instead of plain talk. Misunderstandings can also occur when the doctor uses common words but the patient misinterprets them because they aren't accustomed to their use in a healthcare context. For instance, "Keep your glucose in a normal range." Does that mean store it in the stove?

2. Provide 'care-full' explanations

The quality of your explanations also contributes to positive clinical outcomes and has well-documented effects on patient satisfaction. When an explanation reduces their anxiety, increases their sense of control, and builds confidence in their caregivers, patients are more likely to absorb information, cooperate in their care, and feel less anxious. This frees up energy for their treatment and healing.

Truly great explanations address more than the tasks and actions at hand. They also address the effective domain—the patient's feelings, anxieties, and concerns. These are the elements that have the greatest positive affect on the patient's experience. They make the caregiver's caring nature clear to patients and families.

Make sure you always follow these three rules:

1. **Make your caring intent clear.** While you certainly mean well as you say and do things for patients, the patient might not realize how your actions are in his or her best interest. A "care-*full*" explanation articulates how what you are doing or suggesting is *for the patient's sake.*

2. **Adjust the patient's expectations to be more realistic.** Unrealistic expectations spark anxiety, complaints, and dissatisfaction. A patient may expect test results back in a day or two. When they don't arrive, the patient thinks, *How dare he keep me waiting so long? Why hasn't my doctor called with the results yet?* If you tell people up front how long procedures will take, how much pain they are likely to experience, how

you can help them with it, and when they can expect results, they can adapt accordingly, knowing that their care is progressing as expected and that you want them to feel informed and secure.

3. **Proactively address people's spoken and unspoken anxieties.** Because you have seen many patients going through similar procedures, illnesses, courses of treatment, and emotional swings, you can often anticipate the patient's and family's likely anxieties. Address them proactively, and they will appreciate you for it.

3. Check the patient's understanding

You told them, but did they understand it? Care-full explanations are only effective if they are understood by the person on the receiving end. After inviting patients and families to ask questions and giving them thorough explanations, *check for understanding.* It's not enough to ask if the patient understands—the patient's answer tells you nothing. People are often afraid to admit that they don't understand, or they might not realize they don't understand. And if they say "yes," you then have no confirmation about what they understood.

Check understanding in a way that makes patients comfortable and gets them talking. Find out in a way that's not insulting—tell them you want to know if *you* have been clear, not whether *they* have understood. Use open-ended questions, such as:

- "Many people are confused by this explanation. What's your understanding of the main points?"

- "I've said a lot, and I'm concerned that I might not have been clear. What is your understanding of the most important things to do once you get home?"

- "So much information can be overwhelming. What questions do you have at this point?"

- "When you're not feeling well, it can be hard to concentrate on the details. What's your understanding of the next steps?"

- "Would you mind repeating back to me what you understand to be the next steps? This is complicated, and I want to make sure I included everything important."

An explanation is incomplete until you respectfully make sure it hit the mark.

4. Reinforce your verbal explanations with other media

Most important to the patient: care plan instructions. Patients appreciate complete written instructions when they leave your office. For the main conditions you treat, preprint instructions or make a checklist that you can quickly fill out. Have your staff field-test them with patients to identify incomplete or unclear information. For instance, if you instruct a patient to take a certain medication three times a day, should they take the medication at mealtime, on an empty stomach, or before bed?

The physician who preempts patients' feelings of insecurity and uncertainty by effectively explaining and ensuring comprehension stands out as competent, patient-centered, and caring.

Engage patients in their own healthcare decisions

While some people continue to view physicians with deference and accept advice without question, increasingly, patients want and expect to know their options and make their own decisions. Also, there is increasing research showing that engagement in decisions leads to a reduction in symptoms and better patient outcomes.

But patient engagement is not a simple matter. Some physicians believe that patient engagement consumes time that they don't have because they need to convey so much more information and hold discussions until the patient feels committed to one decision or another. However, research does not bear this out. Instead, while the discussion of information takes time, the greater commitment of the patient to his or her care plan and adherence to it that results from engagement ends up saving time in the end.

Another obstacle to shared decision-making and patent participation is the fact that many physicians prefer to maintain an imbalance of power with their patients and somehow communicate this. As a result patients are reluctant to share their preferences, and the physician is convinced that they didn't want to participate after all.

These days, for the sake of patients' satisfaction with their physician and optimal health outcomes, engaging patients and sharing decision-making are crucial. The committed physician takes steps and builds skills to understand patient preferences and to empower them and encourage their active participation.

When you engage patients in true dialogue and mutual understanding about their concerns, needs and preferences, you produce better outcomes. But that's not all. Patients will perceive you as helpful, respectful, and responsive, and they appreciate you for it. Patients believe you're on their side. Use the physician self-check in Figure 8.3 to gauge the effectiveness of your communication skills.

FIGURE 8.3   Physician Communication Self-Check

In my communication with my patients and families, do I . . .	Always	Most of the time	Sometimes	Never
1. Realize that eliciting the patient's experience and perspective will make me more, not less efficient?				
2. Pause and listen without interrupting after I ask a question?				
3. Listen for information, feelings, preferences, and expectations?				
4. Check my understanding of what the patient seems to be thinking and feeling?				
5. Explain my positive intent and how what I am doing or saying is for the patient's sake?				
6. Ask open-ended questions to get the person talking?				
7. Make it comfortable for the patient to ask questions?				
8. Elicit information about the patient's cultural context, so I can provide better care?				
9. Check the patient's understanding of key information, options, plans, and his or her responsibilities?				
10. Mean it when I encourage the patient to ask questions?				
11. Make a concerted effort to share decision-making with my patients to respect their choices and influence more positive outcomes?				
12. Empower them with easy-to-understand sources of information so they can make wise decisions on their own behalf?				

Overcoming Cultural Barriers

Let's say you're sharing a test result with a patient, and you give them a thumbs-up. You mean "all's well." But a thumbs-up in many cultures means something very different; it is considered to be a sexual insult or proposition. Consider also eye contact. If an American avoids eye contact, it often reveals discomfort or untruthfulness. In Asian cultures, however, looking away can signify respect.

Every individual and family you serve arrives with a unique set of health beliefs and practices that shapes their perceptions of you as a provider and affects how they will respond to care. To reach and involve the patient more completely, it is so important to know his or her personal context, viewpoints, and goals. Without this, how can you ensure that they understand your approach? How can you obtain truly informed consent? How can you strengthen the likelihood that they will adhere to treatment and follow-up as needed? How can you earn their trust and confidence and a positive evaluation of the experience?

Individual and cultural differences shape a person's:

- Thinking about good versus poor health

- Interpretations of symptoms

- Beliefs about the etiology of their health issues

- Ideas about preventive care and appropriate treatments

- Beliefs about their own ability to influence their health status

- Expectations of their physicians

Ask, learn, and accommodate

By asking artful open-ended questions, you can learn important, culturally influenced information that will enable you to tailor your consultation, decisions, relationship, and communication to the individual patient.

By taking some time to gain *general* knowledge of the health beliefs and practices of the cultural groups you serve, you will then be in a good position to tailor your inquiry to the *individual*. Ask questions that inform you about the patient's cultural context.

It is always dangerous to make assumptions. Although cultural patterns differ from one group to another (whether by generation, age, race, gender, country of origin, socioeconomic status, sexual orientation, or personality factors), there are also significant differences between individuals in the same reference group. While it is known that African Americans are more likely to have high-blood pressure than are Caucasians, it doesn't mean that your African

Cultural factors to investigate

- Self-care strategies
- Beliefs about the origins of disease
- Body image
- Contraceptive knowledge
- Family rituals and crisis management
- Child-rearing practices
- Gender roles
- Use of "chemical comforters," herbs, and other self-medicating approaches
- Religious beliefs with implications for the handling of health and illness
- Social networks and support
- Dietary patterns
- Perceptions of elders
- Noncompliance (nonadherence) issues, which are often based on different beliefs or values
- Patterns related to expressing and handling pain
- Desire for information
- Decision-making
- Gaining trust
- Misunderstandings other caregivers have had based on cultural differences and what they learned from these

American patient has high blood pressure. Knowing about cultural patterns helps you to see possibilities, but it is not predictive when applied to an individual from that group.

The more constructive approach for healthcare providers is to observe, read cues, and above all ask questions to find out about an individual and the meaning he or she attaches to the present situation.

Could some of your patients be different, not difficult?

We all have cultural biases, and for providers, these biases tend to surface in moments of frustration or when we feel like we're not communicating well. Think of the patients you serve. Do any ruffle your feathers because they:

- Don't speak English as well as you do?
- Defer decision-making power to other family members?
- Withhold pertinent information, such as alternative health treatments or pain levels?
- Are too dependent on family?
- Demand too much of your time?
- Wait too long to come in for care?
- Agree to adhere to your advice and then fail to follow through?

How do you deal with these issues? Respond with genuine curiosity, acceptance, and respect. Ask questions so you can learn more and know what to expect and how to engage the patient's family or interpreters, if that can help.

Often, cultural barriers can be overcome by simply asking the right questions and dedicating the time and effort to understanding the patient. Consider this expanded list of helpful questions (Figure 9.1).

Learn cultural relativism

A culturally competent approach to patient care is based on *cultural relativism*. Instead of viewing patients' health behaviors and expectations according to the standards of *your* culture, you view them according to standards consistent with *their* values.

FIGURE 9.1   Interview Questions for Diverse Patients

Category	Questions
1. Pathophysiology	What do you call your problem? What name does it have? How does it work?
2. Symptoms	What does it do to you? What do you feel?
3. Etiology	What caused it? Why has it happened to you? Why now?
4. Diagnosis	How much do you know about it? What do you think went wrong?
5. Prognosis	How severe is it? How long do you think it will last? What are you most worried about with this?
6. Social assessment	Is there someone, in addition to you, with whom you want us to discuss your medical condition? Who can you talk to about your health? Do you know anyone else who has this same problem, and if so, what happened with him or her?
7. Authority and con-sent	Is there someone other than you involved in your healthcare decisions? Who would need to consent in order for you to have a procedure?
8. Roles	What do you expect from me? What can I expect from you?
9. Treatment	What do you think will make your problem go away? What kind of results are you looking for? What kinds of traditional health remedies do you use or are you thinking of using?
10. Taboos	Are there certain healthcare procedures and tests that your culture prohibits? Are there things that make you nervous about our healthcare system?
11. Past experiences with healthcare	Please tell me about your experiences with healthcare in your native country. How often each year did you see a healthcare provider before you arrived here? What differences have you noticed between care you received in your country and the care you receive here?
12. Communication preferences	What languages are spoken in your home? What language or languages do you understand and speak?
13. Self-care	What have you done so far to treat this? How do you think your approach is working? What are your thoughts about continuing it?
14. Self-efficacy	How confident are you that you can do what's needed in order to recover?

Patients want their differences to be recognized, understood, and respected. Examined and treated within their own cultural context, they experience a higher quality of care, and you can achieve more effective clinical outcomes.

Consider these additional tips:

- When possible, interview and assess patients in the target language or via appropriate use of bilingual/bicultural interpreters.
- Write or obtain instruction sheets and handouts and provide these to patients to reinforce your spoken explanations.
- Effectively use community resources to identify translators and people who might educate you and your team about cultural factors that might affect your patients who belong to that group.
- Ask the patient to repeat back information provided so you can check their understanding.
- Clearly communicate expectations.
- Speak slower, not louder.
- When appropriate, use drawings and gestures to aid communication.
- Make no assumptions about education level or professionalism.
- Avoid using phrases such as "you people," which many consider to be culturally insensitive. A reflective approach is useful. Examine your own biases and expectations to understand how these influence your interactions and decision-making

10

Difficult Encounters and Hard Conversations

No doubt, there are times you feel frustrated or annoyed with a patient or a patient's family member. Perhaps the patient is pressing you for more time than you can give. Or the patient asks for medication that you know he or she doesn't need. Or you want to raise a touchy issue with a patient about his or her diet, smoking, or lack of follow-through with self-care.

How you handle strained interactions can make or break the patient experience during a difficult encounter. It can also make or break your peace of mind in the course of your busy day.

In difficult encounters, caring communication goes a long way toward easing patient frustration and anxiety. There are four keys to handling difficult encounters in a way most likely to reduce the heat and win patient cooperation.

1. Do all you can to satisfy the patient

First, see if you can responsibly accommodate the person's request or offer options that ease the situation. When people are resistant or upset, listen carefully to determine possible options for correcting the problem. If at all possible, get creative and figure out how to do what they want unless it is illegal, unethical, or in your professional opinion not in their best interest.

2. Tell the truth

If you can't accommodate what a patient wants, say so directly. Always tell patients the truth and do it quickly. Don't beat around the bush. Make your position clear in a small number of words. For instance:

- "I'm not comfortable doing that."
- "I am not able to do that."
- "I am not willing to do that."
- "That's not an option."

3. Be direct but caring

While being direct, be clear that you care. Mix your message with expressions of caring using these caring communication skills:

- Stay tuned in and present to the person.
- Acknowledge the person's feelings. "I realize this may be inconvenient for you."

- Show your caring nonverbally. Look kindly and concerned, not harsh or irritated.

- Explain your positive intent and use the words "for you." As in, "I want what's best for you." Or "I want to do the right thing for you."

- Offer a blameless apology. "I'm sorry it's frustrating for you."

4. Be a 'caring broken record'

Once you've done all you can and have communicated your caring, if the patient continues to resist, insist, or persist, hold your ground with the "caring broken record." Don't address each of the person's arguments or excuses. Kindly repeat yourself. Hold your ground by repeating your message, sometimes over and over again, and always couched in caring and sympathetic language. You can vary the language so you don't sound irritated or harsh, but make the same point each time.

Here's how this might sound. Let's say a parent, Mrs. Macklin, arrives with her son Jimmy for his appointment. She also has her two daughters Susie and Lizzie in tow. Mrs. Macklin asks Dr. Miller to examine them too. First, Dr. Miller tries to accommodate them. "I want Lizzie and Susie to get the attention they need. I didn't expect to see them right now, but I think we can fit them in. Will you please stop at the desk and register them? Then we'll fit them in as soon as possible. It could take up to 30 minutes. Or would you prefer to make an appointment for another day?"

But if Dr. Miller can't accommodate them without wreaking havoc on the appointment schedule, then he can say "no" by repeating his message like a caring broken record:

Dr. Miller: I want Susie and Lizzie to get the care they need. Right now we have a room full of patients with appointments who are waiting to be seen. Since I didn't expect to see Susie and Lizzie today, I'm asking you to make another appointment for them. I'm afraid it wouldn't be fair to keep everyone else waiting.

Mrs. Macklin: But they're here now, and it would be so great if you could see them now.

Dr. Miller: I wish I could make this convenient for you. It's just that I want to give Susie and Lizzie my full attention, and I don't have time now without making other people wait who have appointments. I'm asking you to make an appointment for each of them so I can give them my undivided attention. I really appreciate your understanding, Ms. Macklin.

The caring broken record works in a wide variety of difficult encounters, including sharing of bad news. You couch your main message in explicit expressions of empathy and caring and repeat it in the face of resistance.

The fact is, your way of handling difficult interactions with patients, families, and coworkers has a powerful effect on everyone's satisfaction. By handling tough situations and hard conversations with straightforwardness and caring, you can retain the patient's goodwill, achieve optimal clinical results, and reduce your own stress so you can leave with a "good tired" feeling at the end of your day.

Caring and Helpful Office Staff

Because every member of your practice team plays a part in the patient experience, the Consumer Assessment of Healthcare Providers and Systems survey, the Medical Group Management Association survey, the Press Ganey survey, the Massachusetts Health Quality Partners survey, and other medical practice patient satisfaction surveys include several questions about office staff performance. For your office team to have a consistently positive effect, staff members need to be efficient with your business practices and have a patient-centered focus—helpful, responsive, and caring in their interactions with patients and families.

By strengthening the four pillars of a patient-centered staff, you can ensure that your office staff members not only know their job tasks but also excel in their interactions with patients and families.

The four pillars of a patient-centered staff

1. Leadership vision and behavior, commitment, and modeling
2. Hiring and accountability
3. Employee training and difficult situations support
4. Feedback, focus, and continuous improvement

On the accompanying CD-ROM you'll find a variety of tools related to the material in Section III, including:

- Great customer service: Hiring tools
- Accountability tools
- Employee recognition tools
- Flyers/posters that raise staff awareness
- Tools for handling delays and waiting
- Tools that ease strain related to insurance and money
- Scripts for difficult situations

Pillar 1: Leadership Vision and Commitment

As a leader intent on providing quality patient experiences, it's important to establish and communicate your personal patient-centered vision for your practice. This vision and your personal commitment to it provide the context for expectations and initiatives to enhance the patient experience to fulfill that vision.

As an example, a physician leader in a large primary care practice in Philadelphia posted this letter in a frame on the office wall:

"Statement of Committment"

"Taking great care of our patients and families and helping them stay as healthy as possible is the reason we're here. I want this practice to put our patients and families first. I want everyone, and I know this starts with me, to make a personal connection to the people we serve, to listen to them, to partner with them in their care, and to meet their needs in a manner that is not only competent, but also timely, responsive, and compassionate. I know this is not easy, because we have demanding, stressful jobs. To accomplish this, we need each other's teamwork, cooperation, and support. Together we can make the patient and family experience great and earn widespread respect, a wonderful reputation, and a loyal patient following."

If you haven't already done so, establish your statement of commitment. Think this through and make this a *personal* statement. Be clear and explicit. Consider these questions to crystallize your commitment statement:

- What are you committed to achieving in terms of patient-centered care and patient satisfaction?
- Why are you committed to this? Who benefits and how do they benefit?
- How can you convey the message with empathy and understanding (e.g., "I realize it's not easy because . . .")?

This commitment statement should be one that you repeat often. It is your personal bottom line and the reason why you are going to persist in expecting every member of your staff to meet the highest standards of communication and service.

Positive role-modeling

Visibly use your power as a role model in your interactions with your staff, your patients, and their families. Exemplify courtesy, caring, and compassionate communication in your interactions not only with patients and families, but also with every member of your staff. Greet people by name and with eye contact and a smile every day. Warm up the climate in your practice with your own gracious behavior and person a presence.

As leader, you set the example for every person on the staff. If you don't acknowledge a person, that person is likely to think, "Wow, did you see that? And he expects US to greet people warmly!" Your staff members look to you for leadership, and they will resent double standards—expectations you have of them that you do not live up to yourself.

How do you think you're perceived by your staff in routine situations? Consider the assessment in Figure 11.1.

Your staff members look to you as an example, so practice what you preach— or, as Ghandi said, "Be the change you want to create."

FIGURE 11.1   Role-Modeling Assessment

(Instructions: Check "Strength" if you agree with a statement. Otherwise, check "Room for improvement.")

Strength	Room for improvement	Statement
		1. I warmly greet each person on my staff when I first see him or her each day.
		2. As I pass people in the hall, I acknowledge them with a smile and eye contact.
		3. When someone comes to my office, I give a warm welcome before delving into the business at hand.
		4. When a member of my staff appears upset, I express concern.
		5. I make sure to communicate that I care about my staff.
		6. I say "thanks" to individuals often, making it clear that I don't take their work and dedication for granted.
		7. When I'm stressed or frustrated, I'm careful to avoid taking it out on my staff.
		8. I avoid making negative comments about patients to my staff.
		9. When I notice that a member of my staff needs help, I offer to pitch in.
		10. When a staff member makes a suggestion, I listen to him or her and appreciate that the staff member spoke up.
		11. When I'm annoyed with a staff member, I find a way to address it directly in a tactful way.
		12. I deliver on my promises: I arrive when I say I will. I return calls when I say I will. And when I can't, I let people know.
		13. I say goodbye to staff members as I leave the office or as I see them leaving.
		14. I encourage my staff to speak up when they are having a problem, even if the problem is with me.

FIGURE 11.1   Role-Modeling Assessment (cont.)

		15. I treat every person on my staff with respect.
		16. I express my appreciation to people when they have had a particularly challenging day.
		17. When someone leaves my office, I wish him or her a warm and appreciative goodbye.
		18. I give my staff feedback on their performance.
		19. I compliment my staff members on their style when I think it's effective.
		20. I support events and actions that are morale boosters for my staff.

Pillar 2: Hiring and Accountability

Effectiveness in today's medical practice requires more than technical ability to perform the tasks in the job. Healthcare is in essence a service industry, and every employee must demonstrate key customer service skills. When you hire people who have the ability to communicate with clarity and caring, you can rely on them, they will hit the ground running, and you'll have fewer headaches down the road.

If you don't have a systematic approach to screening job candidates when you have staff openings, consider installing the highly effective "behavioral interviewing" approach. When you screen for service competencies using behavioral interviewing, you will be more likely to pick competent people who are also a good fit with your practice's priority of a great patient experience.

What is behavioral interviewing? It is a methodical, consistent process for screening and selecting candidates for any position based on the premise that past performance is the best predictor of future performance. Instead of asking hypothetical questions or asking the candidate to talk about his or her skills and approaches, you ask the applicant to describe a small number of relevant past experiences in considerable detail.

For instance, if you were to ask the candidate to describe an actual example in the past when he or she handled a very difficult situation with a customer, you ask the question and then probe for the details:

- What was the situation? What happened?
- What did the customer say?
- What did you say? Then what did the customer say?
- How did you feel? How do you think the customer felt? Why did you think that?
- And what did you do?
- And how did the customer react?
- And how did you feel about it afterward?

By learning these details, you *know* how this employee behaves. And you should be hiring for an employee's behavior—not what the employee *thinks* he or she would do in situations like that, but what the employee *actually did*.

Topics that work well for behavioral interview questions include asking the candidate details about a time when:

- The candidate handled an unreasonable request
- The candidate made an improvement that benefited his or her customers

- The candidate was under a lot of pressure and someone asked him or her to stop what he or she was doing to help them out

Only by hearing in rich detail how the candidate performed in a relevant situation in the past can you determine how he or she is likely to handle the demands of the job.

The CD-ROM enclosed with this book includes many more questions, as well as tools that make the hiring process easy and consistent. You'll find:

- Suggested interview questions that screen for specific service and communication competencies
- A list of the best probing questions
- Tactics for controlling the interview and handling sticky situations (e.g., when the candidate talks on and on, is silent, or talks in general terms)
- How to code and take notes
- Tips to consider when making the hiring decision

By hiring for customer-oriented people equipped with emotional intelligence and communication competency, you build a team who share your commitment to a great patient experience and can do their part in making it happen.

Establish clear performance expectations

By adopting and using human resource practices that align with your emphasis on the quality patient experience, you can support and sustain great staff performance.

Human resource practices that support great performance

- Establish a code of conduct for patient-centered service
- Orient new staff to your patient-centered philosophy and office practices
- Include patient-centered behavioral expectations in every employee's job description and performance review
- Provide and institute best-practice scripts for everyday situations
- Ensure that each employee receives performance coaching and feedback

---

Make your expectations explicit to your staff. Some practices do so by engaging patients and staff in identifying important behaviors and building these into a code of conduct. Here's an example:

Sample house rules for patient-centered care and service: Performance expectations for our practice team

1. **Break the ice and the mystique.** Warmly welcome our children and families. Make eye contact and smile; put warmth in your voice; introduce yourself and your role. Find out what people prefer to be called and call them by name often.

2. **Connect and stay connected.** Be present. Focus your full attention on the person you're with. Move to the person's eye level. Tune in completely. Connect. Maintain eye contact. Make the person your sole—and soul—focus.

---

3. **Inform and explain.** Information is power. Share it. Tell customers exactly what they can expect and what will happen next. Invite questions and check for understanding. Apologize for delays.

4. **Make patients and families feel secure during handoffs.** Connect them to the next step in the service process. Prepare them fully. Reduce their anxiety. Build confidence in others on the team.

5. **Anticipate.** You'll often know what people need before they have to ask. Don't wait. Act first. Put children and their families at ease. Offer comforts and options.

6. **Respond quickly.** When children and families are worried and waiting, every minute is an hour. Keep appointments. Return calls. Apologize for delays.

7. **Ensure privacy, confidentiality, and respect.** Watch what you say and where you say it. Protect rights and dignity. Ask permission. Give choices. Knock. Ask customers what they think, feel, and want.

8. **Help each other and you help a child and family.** Just because it's not your job, it doesn't mean you can't help or find someone who can. Pitch in. Communicate directly with one another. Say thanks. Together, we can create a supportive office culture.

9. **Take care on the phone.** Our reputation is on the line. Sound pleasant. Listen with understanding. Help.

10. **Maintain a professional image.** We're part of a long, proud medical tradition. We have a public face and a public importance. Look the part.

Patient-centered behavioral expectations

Every member of your team needs to understand up front the behaviors expected of him or her to contribute to the great patient experience. Team members also deserve to know what's expected of them so they won't be surprised later when they are encouraged to act accordingly and held accountable.

Include statements like these in staff job descriptions:

Job description statement

- Follows the house rules for patient-centered care and service.

- Provides great customer service by consistently employing best practices in everyday interactions with patients and families and also with coworkers.

- Greetings: Makes positive first impressions on your customers by behaving in ways that are warm, welcoming, professional, and helpful.

- Handoffs: When handing off a customer to other people/services, uses words/actions that make the customer feel informed, supported and confident in the people on the receiving end.

- Goodbyes: Makes positive last impressions on customers by saying goodbye in ways that are warm, caring, informative, and professional.

- Complaints: Encourages complaints and listens without being defensive; takes action to make things right.

Also add to job descriptions key elements that are critical in the person's specific role. For instance:

Receptionist

- Greets people warmly, introduces oneself, and calls people by their preferred name
- Updates patients on delays at least every 20 minutes
- Takes initiative to make patients comfortable while waiting
- Maintains composure when dealing with difficult or frustrated people and does not become defensive
- Protects patient confidentiality
- Demonstrates helpfulness and teamwork
- Answers the phone within three rings in a way that makes a positive impression

Provider

- Greets coworkers warmly and by name to create respectful office environment
- Maintains presence with patients and families and gives them undivided attention
- Checks for understanding after giving instructions and suggestions
- Invites "one last question" in order to ensure that patient needs are met

Attach the house rules and job-specific service expectations to each person's job description.

Orient new staff to your patient-centered philosophy and office practices

Provide each new employee with an orientation to your patient-centered philosophy, your code of conduct, and job-specific expectations. If you are orienting more than one person at a time, provide this orientation in a group format. Otherwise, have either the employee's supervisor or a skilled peer provide this orientation.

See to it that you or your designee meet with each new employee and accomplishes each action on the following checklist (Figure 12.1). These actions help your new people succeed in the service aspects of their new position.

Performance review process

With the adage "People respect what management inspects" in mind, integrate service expectations into your performance review form and address the relevant behaviors in your discussions with employees. Integrate the same statements that are in employees' job descriptions. For example, Figure 12.2 outlines a sample assessment of service performance for a practice receptionist.

By clarifying your service expectations and building them into all personnel practices, you give your expectations more support—and more teeth.

Provide and institute best-practice scripts for everyday situations

Every day with every patient, your staff members engage in repetitive communications—when they greet a patient, when they hand patients off to others, and when they say goodbye. They also do other things routinely, such as

FIGURE 12.1   11-Point Orientation Checklist

√ Done	Action	Notes/con-cerns/ fol-low-up/needs
	1. Describe the practice's overall goal of being consistently and distinctively great in service interactions with patients and other customers. Review benefits for patients, families, coworkers, and the practice.	
	2. Make a personal statement that communicates your commitment and enthusiasm for the great patient experience.	
	3. Talk with this new person about who his or her "customers" are. Emphasize the importance of coworkers as customers too.	
	4. Walk through a booklet on your practice's commitment to patient-centered care and service (see the CD-ROM enclosed with this book for an example).	
	5. Present the new employee with all existing scripts specific to his or her position. Make these points: • Following these scripts is key to providing consistently great service. • We have learned from our patients what they want. Staff members were involved in developing and fine-tuning these scripts to meet our patients' needs. • You can use your own words as long as you cover the main message points in these scripts. Performance in accordance with these scripts is a job requirement. It's expected and will be a key part of the annual performance review.	
	6. Give the employee a card with your practice's code of conduct on it. Also provide on such cards any job-specific scripts for great customer service in this employee's particular position.	
	7. Decide on a schedule and approach for helping the new employee to learn to perform using these scripts.	
	8. Assign each new employee a buddy, mentor, or coach who will help him or her meet all expectations and check in and help the new employee troubleshoot problems.	
	9. Communicate that you will personally follow-up with the new person to see how he or she is doing and give support.	
	10. Invite and address questions. Let the employee know you will be happy to help at any point along the way.	
	11. Let the employee know that you're happy to have him or her join the team. Thank the new employee in advance for becoming a role model of *great* service to their customers.	

FIGURE 12.2   Sample Performance Assessment (Receptionist)

Factor	1	2	3	4	5	Comments
Greets people warmly; addresses them by their preferred name						
Explains delays often and apologetically						
Offers options when people are frustrated						
Maintains composure in the face of difficult people						

explaining delays, asking for copays, arranging follow-up appointments, etc. Apart from the content of each interaction, the quality of staff communication during these moment-of-truth situations has a great effect on the patient's experience and his or her perceptions of your practice team.

To make routine communications impressive, staff behavior needs to go beyond courtesy and do what we in healthcare uniquely need to do to reduce our patients' anxiety. Many medical practice teams are applying the customer service mindset from the entertainment and hospitality trades to make service improvements for patients and families.

Although we have certainly learned a lot about the power of improving service quality by design from these other industries, patients and families are not like customers in the tourist and entertainment industry. Customers of Disney World, cruise ships, and luxury hotels want to be there. They're excited and ready for a good time. That's not the case when people go to the doctor. We serve people who are anxious, distressed, and often frightened. The goal of "making people happy" is hardly attainable. Our focus needs to be instead on reducing patient and family anxiety. When physicians and their teams take steps to prevent or reduce patient anxiety, patients appreciate it deeply and conclude that their caregivers really care about them.

The differences between a script for common courtesy and a best-practice script for patients lie in components that are deliberately aimed at relieving anxiety. For example, when a staff member is directing a patient to the lab to get a blood test, she could say, "Before you see the doctor, stop at the lab and get your blood drawn." Is that clear? Yes. Was it said in an offensive way? No. But it was not anxiety-reducing, and it could have and should have been. Consider this alternative approach: "Before you see the doctor, would you mind stepping down the hall to the lab? Dawn is our nurse who will take your blood. She's very good and very gentle." By building the patient's confidence in Dawn, the patient becomes less anxious.

Engage your team in developing or locating and instituting best-practice scripts for everyday routines. Help them achieve greater consistency in effective communication by making explicit the key message points that need to be addressed in routine interactions.

The accompanying CD-ROM includes a potpourri of staff scripts for everyday situations. Involve staff in examining, criticizing, and improving upon them to develop their own best-practice approaches.

Pillar 3: Employee Training and Support

The third pillar that supports staff in providing a great patient experience involves training. Without staff training, you have a normal curve of performance with a select few people behaving in a wonderful way, most people somewhere in the middle, and a select few behaving in an offensive way. While there will always be a normal curve, to enhance the patient experience, the standards need to be raised so that the people at the middle are excellent and the small number of people at the top are actually miracle workers. To help people perform at a higher level, training is a necessity and a great investment.

But training for what? To enhance the patient experience, the answer is really communication and self-management skills. Consider how to:

- Do an impressive greeting and goodbye
- Hand off patients to a coworker so you transfer the trust
- Invite and handle complaints
- Communicate empathy and caring

- Explain difficult topics in a way that patients can understand
- Deal with difficult situations, defusing anger, disappointment, and frustration
- Make patients and families feel like the center of your universe for those precious minutes you're serving them
- Confront patients tactfully when necessary
- Give feedback to a disruptive coworker
- Speak up to a physician in a constructive way
- Manage your time
- Manage your stress

There are seven effective ways to provide training opportunities for your staff:

1. Provide books, articles, CDs, and e-learning programs designed to enhance communication skills. Establish a schedule and sponsor a monthly (free) "lunch and learn," learning cafe or book club in which staff rotate leadership and present a selected reading or skill.

2. Send staff to commercially available training programs. Some practices give every staff member a stipend or tuition reimbursement for job-related training. Others support staff participation in outside programs on an ad hoc business to meet specific needs.

3. Bring training in-house. Through your local hospital or independent training consultants you can fund excellent training programs that can meet your practice's particular needs.

4. Invest in facilitator training for one or more members of your staff so they can provide training within your practice.

5. Create a position for a "training professional." Hire a person to provide training, coaching, and team-building.

6. Set up a buddy or mentor system through which skilled individuals work with others one on one to help them build their skills.

7. Insert short skill briefings or snippets into regular staff meetings so that everyone refreshes their skills together.

The point is that some staff won't demonstrate excellent behavior toward patients, families, and each other unless you invest in their development. If you do make the investment, staff feel greater pride in their work, your patients and families see and feel the difference, and your practice wins respect and loyalty.

Support your staff in difficult situations

While patient and family complaints are inevitable, most patients and family members won't go away mad if your staff handles their complaints caringly and skillfully. On the front line, staff members take the heat when patients and families are frustrated, whether the frustration relates to money and insurance issues, delays and waiting, difficulties getting appointments, selection of the provider, or other slights that trigger patient complaints. Many staff members claim that the physicians in their practice don't understand because patients tend to be nice to their physician even after being difficult with or complaining to others on the staff.

Acknowledge that your staff members face stressful interactions daily, equip them with this effective model for handling a complaint, and devote time in meetings to practice related to common complaints.

The H.E.A.R.T. approach to handling complaints

- Hear the complaint. Listen fully, paying close attention to the patient.
- Empathize. Acknowledge and accept the person's feelings.
- Apologize. Express your regret that the customer had a frustrating experience.
- Respond. Take action to resolve the complaint. Offer options and follow through.
- Thank. Thank the person for speaking up.

Also, dedicate resources—possibly in the form of an improvement team—to developing and implementing process improvements and communication protocols related to commonly frustrating stressors.

Example: Tensions related to insurance and money

The two greatest stressors for American families are health issues and money issues—both central to your interactions with patients. It's no wonder that interactions around these issues are vigorous and emotionally charged. So, on the one hand, you have patients very anxious about money and payment. On the other hand, you have staff who themselves have money concerns and identify with your patients when money is the issue. Also, your front office staff is on the front lines taking the heat of patient anxiety and anger.

The challenge: Recognizing that your practice is after all a business, how can you avoid hurting your patients' feelings or making them angry about paying while maximizing your collections? And how can you support your staff with the latitude and tools that will help them handle money issues with a minimum of frustration?

Perform the quick audit of your current practice featured in Figure 13.1. The items reveal keys to reducing patient anxiety and easing staff stress related to money.

One large group practice in Massachusetts focused on money issues for a six-month period and instituted the following eight guidelines to ease stress about money:

1. Allow no surprises. Use multiple methods to tell and retell patients in advance what to expect regarding payment.
2. Educate and reeducate patients about how the insurance payment process works.
3. Diplomatically collect up front.
4. Offer multiple payment options.
5. Provide staff with training in anger management and in dealing with difficult situations.
6. Don't send invoices for amounts less than $10.
7. Make collections personal.
8. As a last resort, have a physician intervene to calm angry patients.

FIGURE 13.1 Insurance and Money: Quick Audit

Action	Yes	No
We tell people up front what they will be expected to pay, so there are no surprises.		
We make an effort to educate and reeducate our patients about how insurance works.		
When insurance snags arise, people on our office staff willingly offer help.		
We offer many payment options for our patients' convenience.		
Our office staff members are patient and nondefensive when families are frustrated with insurance issues.		
Our office staff members make special arrangements with people who can't pay all at once.		
Our staff members are skilled in explaining copays without making either the practice or insurance companies look bad.		
Our staff members demonstrate respect for patients and families regardless of their ability to pay.		

For details about each of these eight strategies including sample fact sheets and scripts for employees, see the accompanying CD-ROM.

The more you can do to prevent and ease staff stress in the face of patient frustration and complaints, the more satisfied your patients will be, and you'll also be more likely to retain talented staff.

Pillar 4: Feedback, Focus, and Continuous Improvement

Help staff members see your practice as others see it. Regular feedback from patients and families helps your entire team stay on course and drives continuous improvement. A mix of methods works best, such as:

- The Consumer Assessment of Healthcare Providers and Systems survey and other patient satisfaction survey data
- Issue-specific mini-surveys (conducted via e-mail or on paper)
- Post-appointment phone interviews
- Patient focus groups
- While-you-wait feedback interviews with patients' companions
- Referral source perceptions
- "Patient drain" tracking to find out why patients leave your practice
- Employee satisfaction surveys
- Meeting agendas that tap employee perceptions of the patient experience
- The good old-fashioned suggestion box
- Complaint tracking to identify recurrent problems needing attention

The fact is, feedback drives improvement. People who choose to be healthcare professionals want to do right by others. In the face of evidence about their performance, most instinctively seek improvement. It's a matter of professional pride.

Dynamic, strong feedback loops are essential. Develop regular routines around displaying and discussing customer feedback, survey results, and focus group information. Feedback loops may include posted charts, a regular column in a practice newsletter, tapes of focus groups (with participants' permission to share these), including one or two frontline staff members in focus groups to take notes and listen to patient feedback directly, and worksheets that feed back a result and ask for reactions and suggestions.

By designing, testing, and using feedback loops conscientiously, you will reap the rich value of listening to patient, family, and staff perceptions of their experiences with your practice.

The accompanying CD-ROM includes details about several tools that are useful in obtaining feedback from patients, family members, and staff, including:

- Walk-throughs of your practice
- Patient and family advisory groups
- Quick report cards
- Staff satisfaction report cards
- Staff meetings to identify staff perceptions of service quality
- On-the-run interviews right after a visit
- Post-visit phone interviews

- Focus groups to tap patient/family perceptions
- Staff interviews with people in waiting areas

Keep patient-centered care and service front and center

With so many competing pressures and priorities, it's not easy to keep the patient experience on the front burner with staff. Yet short-term blasts of attention, even those that produce significant short-term results, don't endure without persistent follow-up and follow-through. The patient experience needs to stay on the front burner or the fire will go out.

Here are five ways to keep up the patient experience momentum with your team:

1. *Share customer feedback.* Share all feedback, both positive and negative, with your staff. Devote time to celebrating positive results and discuss and develop action plans when the results are disappointing.

2. *Address patient experience topics in every meeting.* In just five to 15 minutes, you can maintain the focus in a productive way with agenda items like these:

- Customer feedback analysis
- Quick celebration of positive survey results
- Success story swapping: A time you felt like you made an important difference to one of our customers
- Sharing best practices
- Tough situations clinic (people share a tough interaction and help each other find better ways to handle it)

- Issue analysis and brainstorming: Focus staff on one issue arising from your customer data, then discuss its dynamics and root causes, and brainstorm remedies worth testing

- Recognition opportunities: Structure an easy way for staff to give each other public recognition for making a difference to patients and each other

3. *Provide skill reminders and refreshers.* You can use a mix of flyers, posters, videos, and bytes of coaching to help staff to remember and sharpen caring communication skills. (See the accompanying CD-ROM for a collection of these.)

4. *Target one "breakthrough objective" at a time and go after it.* There are so many factors that affect the patient experience—confidentiality, privacy, respect, noise, empathetic communication, explaining delays, and office amenities. One large group practice in New England instituted a "Standard of the Month" process that focused on one of these factors at a time with the help of posters, briefings on relevant skills in staff meetings, and peer observations. They reported that, by focusing on one standard at a time, they prevented overload, while sparking improvement initiatives. Also, they reported that the shared focus enabled people to see tangible results.

5. *Create an employee appreciation epidemic.* When people feel appreciated, they thrive. In an atmosphere of regard, they work harder and with more energy and dedication to your patients, your practice, and each

other. Institute planned approaches to employee recognition. Plan them so that they really happen, because most employees feel under-appreciated. Use a mix of methods that result in frequent thanks and appreciation for individual as well as team performance: Thank you notes sent to the employee's home, use of "A patient thinks you're great" notepad when a patient praises a specific individual, a stress ball giveaway to everyone for handling a particularly stressful time effectively, and frameable certificates of appreciation to name a few.

Your staff reflects on you and colors the patient experience

Patients spend more time with office staff than they spend with their doctors. Your office staff members create the climate of your practice. The stresses that plague them spill over to patients and families, as well as to interactions with each other. By strengthening the four pillars of a patient-centered staff, you can build a team of people who work together in harmony and who make patients and families feel both less anxious and central to your practice.

Long-Term Approaches to Enhancing the Patient Experience

You have no doubt accumulated many great ideas about how to enhance the patient experience, and hopefully this book has added to your storehouse of possibilities. Yet in the fray of everyday routines, it's not easy to launch and sustain a persistent approach to enhancing the patient experience.

By planning a long-term strategy to enhance the patient experience, you can focus a spotlight on the quality of such experiences and make and sustain positive changes one after another, increasing your practice's value to the patients and families you serve.

Long-term strategies with structure and substance are needed, based on three premises:

1. **Enhancing the patient experience needs to be an ongoing, never-ending process.** As patient expectations soar and consumer scrutiny and competitive forces intensify, "good enough" never is, because the bar keeps rising.

2. **A planned approach is needed to stay on course creating continuous improvements.** The fact is a planned approach with goals, metrics, defined tactics, and an identified squad of internal change agents works far better than a more start-and-stop approach.

3. **Every member of your team can contribute to enhancing the patient experience, and they will find the process stimulating and gratifying.** Strategies to enhance the patient experience help people step back from their everyday routines and become creative for the sake of patients and the team. Because most people who work in healthcare have *chosen* a helping profession, they find it satisfying when they are asked to contribute their energies and ideas to improvement initiatives.

Based on these premises, there is a continuum of long-term improvement approaches that provide options to suit your preferences and your practice's culture and needs. On one end of the continuum is the organic approach to improvement driven by the practice leader's vision for the practice. In the middle is the focused, disciplined, and planned one-change-at-a-time approach. And on the other end is a deliberate, multifaceted culture-building strategy that realigns measurement, accountability, training, recognition and compensation, and communications to support the great patient experience.

Three Approaches to Change

To visualize the differences in approach among the three (of many) strategies along the change process continuum, three examples are described here in greater detail:

1. The organic strategy based on consistent, visionary leadership
2. The feedback-driven rapid cycle improvement strategy
3. The culture-building strategy

The organic approach: Leadership-led continuous improvement

For an example of the organic approach to improving the patient experience, look no further than Randy Cook, MD, an internist with Medical Specialists in Hays, KS. His clear vision for relationship-based patient care built the foundation for creating a quality patient experience that has lasted more than 20 years. Dr. Cook understands what's important to his patients, hires people who deliver quality care, actively learns about best practices and has a "let's try it" approach. Without an explicit, staged improvement plan, Dr. Cook implements improvements in an organic yet consistent manner. His approach is sustainable, because his vision and philosophy are consistent and drive his leadership actions to ensure great patient experiences.

About Dr. Cook

Dr. Randy Cook has been practicing medicine for more than 20 years—specializing in treating diabetes—and has built his practice to more than 4,500 patients, 70% of whom are on Medicare. In addition to three physician partners, Medical Specialists has 12 staff members, including two physician assistants (one of whom is a certified diabetes educator), three RNs, three LPNs, and three front clinic office assistants.

The exceptional patient experience provided by Medical Specialists is grounded first of all in Dr. Cook's relationship-based care philosophy. "Our practice's success is all about building relationships with our patients," he says. "We want our patients to feel known and important to us. We want them to open up to us. We want to ease their anxiety. We want them to ask questions and trust us. We want them to feel safe that we're here when they need us. That's what this work is all about."

In keeping with this philosophy, Dr. Cook leads the practice based on several goals important to him:

- Building and sustaining relationships

- Minimizing patient anxiety

- Easing patients' way through our complex healthcare system

- Building trust that leads to open communication, adherence to care plans, and better outcomes

Over the years, Dr. Cook has instituted a number of practices that now characterize patients' experience with him and his practice.

Personalizing care

During their initial visit, staff members take patients' pictures. The patient's photo goes onto the front of his or her chart, and it is updated as the patient ages. While the practice does use an electronic medical record, each patient's paper chart includes a personal page with the patient's preferred name and personal information such as births, marriages, vacations, milestones, achievements, and hobbies. The patient's picture and preferred name prompt staff members to greet the patient by his or her preferred name upon arrival and at each step in the care process. Dr. Cook uses the notes to connect personally with the patient at the start of each encounter. He points out that it helps him remember past conversations and reconnect to the patient right away. Staff members also know to clip articles from the paper about patients and watch and listen for patient news, so they can add to the chart's personal page.

Dr. Cook also asks the patient about their enthusiasms and he freely shares his own. "I talk about golf, hunting, and fishing, and then the medical problem. It relaxes people," he says. "I'm trying to show I'm a real person. I have a life too. And no matter how I'm feeling, life goes on, and I try to be happy. I want them to feel that their life goes on too and that their happiness matters to me."

When a physician is running more than 10 minutes behind (which is rare), staff members keep patients updated. If the wait will be more than 30 minutes, a staff member calls the patient at home to alert him or her before he or she comes in.

Listening and asking questions

Dr. Cook's personal experience as a patient opened his eyes about the patient experience. "Patients want their physician to listen. And when you listen to their story, you learn what they have," he says. "You have to work a lot less if you sit and listen. It's sad that so many doctors feel they are so pinched for time that they don't have time to listen."

When patients are hospitalized, physician assistants round in the early morning and again with Dr. Cook in the afternoon. In the morning, the physician assistant makes sure all labs and results are up to date for each patient. Then, before the physician assistant and Dr. Cook enter the patient's room, they review labs, x-rays, and progress notes together. They enter as a team and immediately focus their undivided attention on the patient. Dr. Cook sits on the edge of the bed and focuses fully on the patient. He takes care to touch the patient to stay connected and also to learn from the feel of the patient's skin.

"I touch their forehead or hold their hand. I want them to know I'm caring and concerned, and I know this will help me learn more from them too," says Dr. Cook. "Standing at the end of the bed looking like you're trying to get out quickly—that's no way to gain trust. You want the patient to feel your interest in their well-being. Once you do that, it's amazing how they follow your directions, their compliance improves, and their outlook on their health condition improves."

Dr. Cook also takes care to include the patient's family in conversations. And at the end of a visit, Dr. Cook habitually asks, "What questions do you have for me before I leave?"

A harmonious, high-performing team

Years ago, Dr. Cook established explicit behavior standards for his team of employees. He reinforces often that every staff member is important to building and sustaining relationships with patients and their families and that, to maximize their impact, certain behaviors are essential. Team members have defined roles so that patients receive help and support proactively and also can access information and help easily when they need it. For instance, the two people responsible for checkout have as their main responsibility easing each patient's way. At checkout, these people arrange for x-rays, labs, referrals, and consults. They offer directions and maps so patients can get where they're going next.

To foster team-building and recognize the dedication and hard work of his staff, Dr. Cook maintains a kitchen in the office and provides lunch for everyone twice a week.

The 'go-to' doctors

After 23 years, Dr. Cook has a very successful practice, and he attributes his success to putting patients first. A strong philosophy about relationship-based care, a commitment to the great patient experience, and openness to feedback from patients and staff and emerging knowledge of best practices are the underpinnings of Dr. Cook's commitment to provide the exceptional patient experience.

The feedback-driven approach: Rapid-cycle improvement

Terrific for people frustrated by the slow pace of many quality improvement processes, this approach uses patient feedback and patient satisfaction data to drive improvement. Practice leaders meet with everyone in the practice to examine patient feedback and satisfaction data in detail. After discussion and brainstorming, the team pinpoints specific improvement objectives and then identifies subgroups to move forward with one improvement apiece.

These small improvement teams begin making the improvement using the Rapid Cycle Improvement Process developed by the Institute for Healthcare Improvement. The Primary Care Development Corporation in New York City and the John Stoeckle Center for Primary Care Innovation have helped many practices implement and sustain enhancements to the patient experience using this rapid cycle technique.

The steps in this process reflect the Plan, Do, Study, Act (PDSA) model for quality improvement:

- **Plan** a change aimed at quality improvement.
- **Do** the tasks required to implement the change. Test it preferably on a small scale using a small sample of patients and short test period (e.g., a week).
- **Study** the results of the change.
- **Act** to adopt or abandon the change.

This approach has helped many practices implement small improvements. For instance, one practice team was frustrated by disappointing survey scores on the Consumer Assessment of Healthcare Providers and Systems (CAHPS) Clinician and Group Survey question: "On your most recent visit, did this doctor give you easy-to-understand instructions about what to do to take care of these health problems or concerns?"

Since the CAHPS survey was not administered often enough to support a rapid-cycle process, the group develop a short report card with this survey question on it that they planned to administer two days a week to monitor patient perceptions. They then laid out a series of small experiments to see if they could improve perceptions on this factor:

- **Week 1:** The physicians used a "prompt card" as patients' visits would come to an end to prompt the physician to check patients' understanding of their post-visit action steps.
- **Week 2:** The physicians personally filled out a form called "Self-care Actions" with space for medication instructions, activity instructions

and constraints, symptoms needing attention before a follow-up visit, contact information, and the timing for a follow-up visit. The physician gave this to patients before the end of the visit and walked through it with them.

- **Week 3:** The physicians asked patients if they would like an audiotape of their instructions for post-visit care. And if they answered yes, the doctor made that tape as he or she was explaining post-visit self-care suggestions.

- **Week 4:** The physicians wrote patients' names on education materials and highlighted the parts most relevant to their care.

Quick trial runs and feedback lead to a "keep it, fix it, or dump it" decision about each improvement. Then every time new patient feedback became available, the practice team decided to continue to pursue aims already established or start on new ones. The process goes on and on as a long-term, sustainable strategy.

The culture-building approach: Affiliated Pediatric Practices case study

In 2004, dissatisfied with their patient satisfaction scores from their own internal survey as well as a major health plan survey, Affiliated Pediatric Practices (APP) leaders decided to begin what has become the never-ending pursuit of the legendary patient experience. They launched their strategy proactively long before health plans considered making it a contract measure.

Since 2005, APP has measured perceptions of the patient experience by using the well-validated Massachusetts Healthcare Quality Partners (MHQP) survey, which combines the best-performing survey items from the Ambulatory Care Experience Survey (ACES) and the CAHPS survey. It addresses eight domains.

Quality of doctor–patient interactions

1. Communication (how well doctors communicate with patients)
2. Integration of care (how well doctors coordinate care)
3. Knowledge of the patient (how well doctors know their patients)
4. Health promotion (how well doctors give preventive care and advice)

Organizational features of care

5. Organizational access (getting timely appointments, care, and information)
6. Visit-based continuity (seeing your own doctor)
7. Clinical team (getting quality care from other doctors and nurses in the office)
8. Office staff (getting quality care from staff in the doctor's office)

About Affiliated Pediatric Practices

Founded in 1995, The Affiliated Pediatric Practice is now a group of 18 independently owned practices with 85 pediatricians working in 24 community pediatric offices in eastern Massachusetts. This unique collaboration, along with APP's association with the Partners Community Healthcare (PCHI) Network has enabled APP member practices to share successes, insights, and knowledge and develop innovative and award-winning programs that have created a patient-centered practice environment and significantly improved patient care and the patient experience for the families they serve.

To evaluate the progress of their patient experience strategy, APP recently compared their scores on the 2007 MHQP to their scores on the same survey in 2005 and found evidence that their efforts paid off. All APP practices improved in at least one domain. Not only that, but some practices improved in all eight, and more than half improved in at least 50% of the domains.

These positive results were hard-won, because the past two years have been replete with wrenching changes such as implementation of the electronic medical record and, for some practices, unstable physician staffing.

What did APP do to improve patient perceptions of their experience so significantly?

In 2005, APP members began to shine the spotlight on the patient experience by articulating the "legendary" experience as their goal and addressing aspects of it in every venue. Then, over an 18-month period, APP engaged in a long-term process of training and follow-up for all physicians and staff and revamping of human resource practices to align with and support the legendary patient experience.

- Training session one engaged all staff in embracing the goal of the legendary patient experience and established behavioral standards related to everyday situations, especially impressive, anxiety-reducing greetings, handoffs, and goodbyes. It also explored the power of presence or mindfulness in encounters with patients. During the months after this foundation session, APP conducted follow-up campaigns to support practices in actually instituting the higher standards set. The first two months of follow-up focused on implementing great greetings, the next few great handoffs, and finally follow-up supported practice teams in instituting effective closings or goodbyes.

- Training session two helped all staff and physicians strengthen their skills for handling difficult situations, especially by refreshing six "Caring Communication Skills" and also the "Caring Broken Record"—a skill for use when no further accommodations are possible or ethical, and staff members need to hold the line.

- To align human resource practices with the priority on the legendary patient experience, practice managers and supervisors received training and tools to help them hire people with customer service and communication competencies and to incorporate legendary patient experience expectations into job descriptions, new employee orientation, and the performance evaluation process.

- APP then instituted its now annual Patient Experience Summit, during which practices highlight and provide rewards for best practices and achievements for people from all APP practices.

APP leaders assert that these training, standard-setting, and recognition processes have established a common language about the patient experience and also laid a solid foundation of explicit **high** standards for all APP practices, equipping people throughout APP with the communication skills key to providing compassionate care and service.

To build on its success creating a patient-centered culture, APP has also been engaging practice teams in the rapid-cycle improvement process using the Plan-Do-Study-Act improvement model. This model has provided consistent language and tools for making additional improvements in employee and physician performance, as well as access, the office environment, collections, and many other components of the patient experience.

And that's not all:

- Office managers meet every other month and, as one set agenda item, always share at least one best practice in depth.

- Several practices have improved their scheduling methods.

- In 2006, APP formed what has become a very active and helpful Parent Advisory Council, which, regardless of its other agenda, always produces rich feedback and excellent suggestions for improvements to the patient experience.

- To support practices in continuous improvement, consultants from the Stoeckle Center for Primary Care Innovation work with each practice to help it identify practice-specific goals and improvement opportunities and employ effective tools for bringing about these improvements. To support this, several practices are also doing frequent mini-surveys focused on one MHQP domain or another and using the results to drive improvement toward domain-specific goals.

It's no wonder that, in addition to being recognized nationally for exceptional effectiveness in asthma, obesity, and ADHD management, APP won PCHI's prestigious Nesson Award for the patient experience initiative.

As of the 2008–2009 contract between a major payer and APP, patient experience scores on the MHQP have become a contract measure with potential financial consequences. APP doesn't have to scramble in the face of this incentive, because they have internalized the legendary patient experience as a continuing priority over several years. They are intent on persisting with established innovation and improvement processes to make the patient experience in their practices ever better.

Different strokes for different folks

Obviously there is not a single best-practice approach. The long-term continuous improvement strategy that can work for you depends on your priorities, whether there is a burning platform for change in your practice created by patient dissatisfaction, staff turnover, or competitive pressures, and your personal style preference along the continuum from an organic change process on one end to a sequential, orchestrated change process on the other end.

The Exceptional Patient Experience Going Forward

Consumers want more. They want a satisfying total experience with a well-delivered clinical service being only one element. To thrive in a competitive environment with ever-more educated patients and with technology options and Internet services exploding, medical practices must orchestrate *memorable events* for patients and families.

Your product is not only the clinical outcome for the patient, but also the patient's memory of the experiences he or she has with you and your practice. Practices transforming into advanced micropractices and medical homes are finding consumers willing to pay more for the memory and added value of the experiences they find there.

Where are the greatest opportunities to enhance the patient experience even further?

Patient–physician partnerships

As more practices embrace the concepts of patient and family engagement in care, it's becoming clear that patients will judge their experience less by what the physician and medical practice do for them and more by what the physician and medical practice do with them.

The experience of the patient and patient's family can be enhanced by engaging them more actively in evaluating treatment options and results, monitoring and reporting their experiences as they adhere to their care plans, reviewing patient perception data, and collaborating in the design of practice enhancements.

As the patient's role in the healthcare process changes, so will the physician's. Those who are able to adapt quickly and meet the needs of both the new, engaged patient and the traditional patient will have the most success.

Supportive work environment

There are many ways to enhance the patient experience, but it makes no sense to enhance that experience at the expense of your staff. To provide consistently great patient experience, we need to make sure we take care of the people who take care of the people.

Do your staff members have doable jobs? Are your expectations of them achievable? Are there work conditions that motivate them to seek other settings where the grass is greener? Do you have enough staff members or staff role definitions that allow them to successfully serve their customers and support your daily effectiveness?

Some facilities are already located in areas experiencing staffing shortages in one form or another, and as demand for healthcare services rises in the near future, recruiting and retaining staff will be even more essential. Consider some of the following:

- If you have piles of phone messages and can't call everyone back in a timely fashion, your staff takes the heat.
- If your front desk person is expected to answer every call within three rings and simultaneously help people register in person, how can this person help but offend either callers or the people standing expectantly in front of him or her?
- If your systems allow details about patient visits, medical records, and test results to fall through cracks, you staff takes the heat on that too.
- If the physical environment is not conducive to a professional and organized approach to work, your staff will either underperform and cast a shadow on your services or turnover to a degree that causes you perpetual staffing and service headaches.

Pervasive respect

Is respect an overarching theme in your leadership style, your vision for your practice, and your entire team's interactions with both patients and staff?

With escalating pressures of patient volume, competitiveness, patient demands for rapid, personal service, and profitability in a volatile payment environment, stress can cause tempers to flare and personal slights to abound. The exceptional patient experience depends on your showing the way for every person on your team to extend the utmost respect and kindness toward every patient and, sometimes even more difficult, toward each other. And of course, it starts with you.

The patient experience that is reliable, predictable, and consistent requires considerable vision, leadership, team-building, open communication and a willingness to do things differently. The results: A thriving practice with appreciative and loyal patients and a gratified, loyal staff.